TUBERCULOSIS

TUBERCULOSIS

Carol A. Dyer

Biographies of Disease
Julie K. Silver, M.D., Series Editor

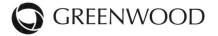 GREENWOOD

AN IMPRINT OF ABC-CLIO, LLC
Santa Barbara, California • Denver, Colorado • Oxford, England

Library of Congress Cataloging-in-Publication Data

Dyer, Carol A.
   Tuberculosis / Carol A. Dyer.
      p. cm. — (Biographies of disease)
   Includes bibliographical references and index.
   ISBN 978-0-313-37211-7 (print : alk. paper) — ISBN 978-0-313-37212-4 (ebook) 1. Tuberculosis. I. Title.
   RA644.T7D88   2010
   616.9'95—dc22   2009044462

ISBN: 978-0-313-37211-7
EISBN: 978-0-313-37212-4

14 13 12 11 10   1 2 3 4 5

This book is also available on the World Wide Web as an eBook.
Visit www.abc-clio.com for details.

Greenwood Press
An Imprint of ABC-CLIO, LLC

ABC-CLIO, LLC
130 Cremona Drive, P.O. Box 1911
Santa Barbara, California 93116-1911

This book is printed on acid-free paper ∞

Manufactured in the United States of America

To my mother, whose love has been the constant in my life.

Contents

Series Foreword

Every disease has a story to tell: about how it started long ago and began to disable or even take the lives of its innocent victims, about the way it hurts us, and about how we are trying to stop it. In this Biographies of Disease series, the authors tell the stories of the diseases that we have come to know and dread.

The stories of these diseases have all of the components that make for great literature. There is incredible drama played out in real-life scenes from the past, present, and future. You'll read about how men and women of science stumbled trying to save the lives of those they aimed to protect. Turn the pages and you'll also learn about the amazing success of those who fought for health and won, often saving thousands of lives in the process.

If you don't want to be a health professional or research scientist now, when you finish this book you may think differently. The men and women in this book are heroes who often risked their own lives to save or improve ours. This is the biography of a disease, but it is also the story of real people who made incredible sacrifices to stop it in its tracks.

Julie K. Silver, M.D.
Assistant Professor, Harvard Medical School
Department of Physical Medicine and Rehabilitation

Preface

Tuberculosis (TB) didn't mean much to me when I was a kid. While it had been a defining feature of my parents' and grandparents' generations, TB was a disease that I had only a vague awareness of. I never worried about catching it and I never knew anyone who had it. For me, TB meant having to have a skin test before I could go to school and hearing stories about people lining up to get chest x-rays in specially equipped vans that were part of a mobile TB screening program. When I was a kid, the thing that I remember the most about TB was the yearly ritual of using Christmas Seals—affixing a decorative stamp to the envelope of every Christmas card we sent to help raise funds for the fight against TB.

I'm sure that I didn't fully understand what TB was at the time, but I do remember how much I looked forward to seeing the new stamp each holiday season. I collected the mail as the holidays drew near and eagerly anticipated the day the new seals would finally arrive. I always loved the picture that decorated it—it was merry and festive, the image of a jolly Santa Claus or a sleigh full of toys. I loved licking the back of the Christmas Seal, even though the glue didn't taste very good, and sticking one on each envelope—my sisters and I used to fight over who got to do it. But Christmas Seals didn't mean TB to me; they meant Christmas. Even though I didn't recognize the importance of TB, I remember being

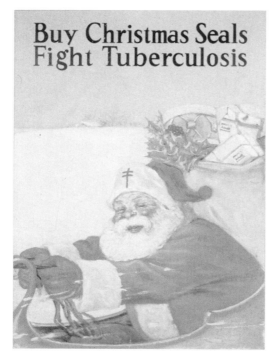

The Christmas Seal for 1927. Christmas Seals are affixed to the packages in Santa's sack, and the Christian double-barred cross is on the brim of his hat. This cross is the anti-TB emblem. Reprinted with permission ©2009 American Lung Association. For more information about the American Lung Association or to support the work it does, call 800-LUNG-USA (800-586-4872) or log on to www.LungUSA.org.

proud that my family participated in the cherished annual tradition of donating money to the American Lung Association. I don't recall the exact year that we stopped using Christmas Seals—the American Lung Association just celebrated 100 years of Christmas Seals to fight lung disease, so they didn't go away—but the fervor over TB did. The magic bullets of medicine, the antibiotics, could now cure TB and it was assumed that this disease would disappear as polio had earlier. The doctors and scientists had finally figured it all out and TB, along with my beloved Christmas Seals, were just going to be memories. Or so everyone thought.

Fast forward several years, and TB is back with a vengeance. The bacteria that cause TB have existed since the beginning of time and in spite of miraculous medical advances, TB has managed to survive and it kills new victims every day. Even though it dropped off the radar for several decades, today TB rages on at epidemic levels in some parts of the world. It is not a disease that frequently makes the headlines in the United States because TB is usually kept at bay in wealthy, developed nations with access to health care and disease prevention. Does this mean that TB is not important to people who live in the United States or other countries where it doesn't occur at high rates? No, it doesn't. TB is an infectious disease—anyone, anywhere can get it. While it is true that TB is an opportunistic infection that takes advantage of conditions in developing nations and things like poverty, HIV, and homelessness, no one is fully immune to it.

This book is neither a medical text nor a history book. It is the biography of TB—the life story of a disease with a long and destructive past and an actively devastating present. The medicines that can cure TB have been available for a long time, but it still remains one of the leading causes of death from infectious disease in the world. This book tells the story of TB. It explains how a person catches the germ and how it can progress to an active disease. It tells the tale of the early medical practices that were used to treat the dreaded disease, and it celebrates the discovery of the real cause and a real cure. The story of TB is an epic—the people who were affected by it and those who helped to unravel its mysteries are described. However, the most important plotline of this story, the one that underpins every other aspect of the chronicle, is the fact TB has endured and it continues to destroy. How is this possible?

Today, the frontline of the fight against TB is in developing nations where medical personnel and health care systems struggle to reach and treat the millions of people who are affected. Success will require widespread efforts on many fronts and participation at every level—individual, community, national, and international. It is my hope that by reading this book, an appreciation of how TB occurred in the past and an understanding of why it continues to occur in the present will encourage greater awareness to help ensure that its future is short and limited. TB didn't mean much to me when I was a kid—I hope it will come to mean something to you. TB is a global problem that has relevance to every person on this planet whether it occurs in your neighborhood or not. To quote the World TB Day slogan from 2008 "TB anywhere is TB everywhere."

ACKNOWLEDGMENTS

This book would not have been possible without Annie-Laurie, whose help and guidance gave me the courage to believe that this would one day be a reality. I feel a special pride in having been able to rely on my daughter's editorial expertise and good judgment throughout this effort. Special thanks to Bill Sterling for generously contributing his graphic design knowledge and talent. I would also like to thank Julie Silver for her encouragement and support. Her accomplishments are an inspiration and I am forever grateful for the opportunity she has given me.

Introduction

Tuberculosis (TB) has been known by many names throughout its long tenure on this earth—as *phthisis* in ancient Greek medical traditions, as consumption to describe its attendant wasting as the body is consumed by disease, and eventually by the name we know it as today. Calling this ancient disease by the name tuberculosis was homage to the field of science and medicine for recognizing that germs were responsible for disease and for discovering the specific bacteria that caused TB. Terms steeped in description and history instead of science became passé as the world embraced new medical terminology and hope that a cure for TB was possible.

It would take some time (more than 50 years), but the hope was eventually realized when the antibiotics that could cure TB were discovered and developed. The medical establishment decreed that the problem of TB was solved and the public was more than ready to agree. TB, however, did not cooperate with the experts—as soon as an antibiotic that could kill M. *tuberculosis* was found, this resourceful bacteria demonstrated its spectacular evolutionary prowess and quickly became resistant to the treatment. One drug was not enough to stop TB, but as additional antibiotics were discovered it was determined that combination treatment with several different antibiotics could outmaneuver the bacteria. When prescribed treatments are taken for a long enough period of time, TB is a curable disease. But throughout the world, TB persists in spite of the cure. There must be more to this story than microbiology, the principles of infectious disease, and effective antibiotic treatment.

Beyond the laboratory and in concert with its relationship with a human host, TB exists in a broader socioeconomic and political environment. René Jules Dubos (1901–1982) was a microbiologist, pathologist, and environmentalist who devoted most of his professional life to the study of microbial diseases. He confronted TB through both pioneering professional work and devastating personal loss. Using his unique understanding of the field of microbiology and the process of disease, Dubos was able to merge his scientific theories with a growing social awareness that carried his ideas far beyond the laboratory. Recognizing that man and both good and bad microbes coexist in the world, Dubos knew that bad microbes were not inherently destructive to humans and that they could live in a dormant state in the body for long periods of time, causing no damage. From this knowledge, he reasoned that other forces must also be at work to enable bacteria to begin the process of disease. By applying his insights to TB, Dubos decided that the destructive power of M. *tuberculosis* must not be related to any specific geographic, climatic, or racial factor since the bacteria existed everywhere but were only selectively destructive.

As his interest in health grew beyond the relationship between the individual and disease, Dubos began to observe how environmental factors contributed to the power of disease. What dynamics contributed to a situation in which a disease was able to overwhelm a whole country or even a continent? Believing that global problems are irretrievably linked to local circumstances and choices, Dubos coined the phrase "Think Globally, Act Locally" to explain his position that world problems, including diseases, can only be addressed through consideration of the ecological, economic, political, and cultural factors that exist in local surroundings.

In his 1952 book *The White Plague: Tuberculosis, Man, and Society*, Dubos prophetically proclaimed that "tuberculosis is a social disease, and presents problems that transcend the conventional medical approach." He was among the first to understand the danger of treating the disease while ignoring the social context in which it existed. Dubos recognized that exposure to the bacteria that caused TB was more apt to result in disease if certain social and economic factors were present; poverty, poor sanitation, overcrowding, inhumane living conditions, and malnutrition may create a population that is vulnerable to disease. The social environment establishes the likelihood of developing disease and, in turn, the disease goes on to leave a footprint on the society in which it develops—this is the nature of TB. The philosophy of a socio-environmental context for TB has never been more relevant than it is today.

In the 1980s, after many decades of decline, the world experienced a dramatic resurgence in the global prevalence of TB. This marks the beginning of the modern era of TB. Increasing rates of TB in many developed countries, including the United States, caused public health officials to closely examine the global state of the disease. What they found was shocking—TB was out of control across most of the poorest regions of the world, especially in Central Africa and South Asia. In 1993, the World Health Organization took the extraordinary step of declaring a global health emergency in light of epidemic rates of TB incidence and death. Since 2004, renewed TB control efforts and increased worldwide awareness of the crisis have contributed to a slowing of the epidemic, but major obstacles still prevent the worldwide elimination of TB. True to the philosophies of René Jules Dubos, socioeconomic issues such as poverty, HIV, homelessness, and biological factors have created treatment-resistant strains of disease that allow TB to survive.

Ultimately, global TB control will depend on understanding the environment in which it thrives and developing ways to manage the factors that breed it. No singular strategy is sufficient to quell the continuing occurrence of TB; a multifaceted approach that respects biological facts, recognizes individual needs, and promotes social well-being is essential. The guiding principles of TB control must be available to all people regardless of socioeconomic status, race, ethnicity, gender, and age. Access to health care and effective treatment, programs to enhance treatment adherence, widespread use of preventive measures, and supportive services will ease the impact of TB on even the poorest communities of the world. Attention to the character of TB and the social factors that promote it allow appropriate services to be concentrated in appropriate places. In the end, history will regard the eventual conquest of this ancient enemy as a comprehensive effort that required much more than medical expertise. True to the ethics espoused by Dubos many years ago, global TB control will ultimately be accomplished by integrating a broad biological and medical knowledge into a social consciousness that embraces the individual and community.

1

Tuberculosis: Contagion and Cause

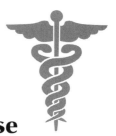

In spite of the fact that tuberculosis (abbreviated TB for tubercle bacilli—the name of the microorganism that causes TB) is a treatable and curable disease, it is currently the second most common cause of death from infectious disease in the world. This blatant contradiction seems to invite an obvious inquiry—if doctors know how to cure TB, why is it still such a deadly problem? Like TB itself, the answer to this question is complicated, multifaceted, and extremely relevant to the current state of health around the world.

TB has existed since the beginning of time. Its profile and history have confounded science and society throughout the ages. The medical tools now exist to make TB a disease of the past, but it still flourishes in places where poverty thrives and health care systems are inadequate and inefficient. TB is a traitor and a scavenger—it sneaks in and lies in wait, it can change itself in order to survive, and it bullies the weak and the poor. Understanding the relationship between the physical and social aspects of TB first requires knowledge of the disease.

THE MYCOBACTERIUM TUBERCULOSIS

Bacteria are round, spiral, or rod-shaped single-cell microorganisms that typically live in soil, water, organic matter, or the bodies of plants and animals. They are individual living systems that are too small to be seen without the aid of a microscope, but they are capable of reproduction, growth, and reaction to stimuli. To organize these microorganisms within the field of biology, bacteria have traditionally been classified by name and grouped on the basis of their features, such as cell structure, cellular metabolism, or cellular components. Beyond this traditional system, modern classification emphasizes the molecular characteristics of bacteria; because information about genetics is constantly being updated, bacterial classification remains a changing and expanding field. The vast majority of bacteria are harmless to human beings because the immune system provides protection against them. The immune system is the bodywide network of cells, tissues, and organs that produce a defensive response to protect the body against invading organisms. In some cases, an immune response against bacteria is not needed and a few types are actually beneficial to the human system. However, some bacteria, like the kind that cause TB, are harmful to people and under the right conditions, despite a fight from the immune system, they can cause contagious and deadly diseases.

The bacteria that usually cause TB in humans have the scientific name *Mycobacterium tuberculosis* (M. *tuberculosis*). Mycobacteria are from the family called Mycobacteriaceae. They are aerobic microorganisms, which mean that they need oxygen in order to grow and reproduce, and they are pathogenic, which means that they are capable of causing disease. The most common and important mycobacterial organisms are the bacteria that cause TB in humans, but other mycobacteria are also able to cause disease in animals and people. For example, *Mycobacterium avium* causes a TB-like illness that is especially prevalent in people who have AIDS, and *Mycobacterium leprae* is the cause of leprosy, a disease characterized by disfiguring skin lesions. *Mycobacterium bovis* (M. *bovis*) causes TB in cows, a form of the disease that can be passed to humans. Bovine TB was once an important cause of TB in children who became exposed to it by drinking milk that contained the bacteria. In most developed countries, cattle are now inspected for disease and milk is heated to kill the bacteria before it is consumed. Bovine TB has become rare; it currently causes only a small percentage of TB cases worldwide.

TB begins when people inhale airborne M. *tuberculosis*. When TB bacteria are inhaled by a healthy person, the immune system is usually strong enough to defend the body and the bacteria remain harmless, producing no infection or subsequent disease. If, however, the bacteria are more powerful than the response produced by the immune system to stop the attack, infection begins and all-out disease may follow. TB infection usually affects the lungs, producing a kind of TB called pulmonary TB. Less frequently, TB infection moves from damaged lung tissue through the bloodstream and affects other parts of the body, like the kidneys, spine, or brain. TB that does not affect the lungs is called extra-pulmonary TB, and since TB must be spread from one person to another through the air, this type of the disease is usually not contagious.

M. *tuberculosis* bacteria are rod-shaped and fairly large compared to other bacteria, measuring two to four micrometers in length and 0.2 to 0.5 micrometers in width. The cell wall structure of M. *tuberculosis* is unique; it is composed of peculiar fatty substances that form a shell around it. This type of cell wall can make the treatment of infection complicated because it can work as a barrier to the drugs that are used to cure it. This may be one of the reasons that TB is a stubborn infection that can resist the drugs used to treat it and it may help to explain why TB can cause such severe disease.

In spite of the cellular characteristics that make M. *tuberculosis* bacteria tough to control, most TB can be successfully treated using combinations of powerful antibiotic medicines. Antibiotic drugs fight bacterial infections by either killing the bacteria that cause the infection or preventing them from reproducing. Effective TB treatment involves the use of several antibiotics for an extended period of time, usually six to nine months. Multiple antibiotics are needed to treat TB because tubercle bacilli are very adaptable and they rapidly become immune to

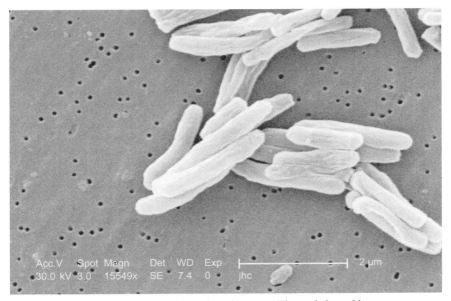

A highly magnified view of M. *tuberculosis* bacteria. This rod-shaped bacterium is between 2 and 4 micrometers long and 0.2 to 0.5 micrometers wide. Courtesy of the Centers for Disease Control and Prevention.

the effect of a single drug. When two or more antibiotics are used at the same time, each drug helps prevent the bacteria from becoming resistant to the other drugs and increases the chance that the bacteria will be susceptible to treatment. If TB is treated with the right combination of drugs for a long enough period of time, the infection can be cured.

However, M. *tuberculosis* is a resilient and adaptable germ—it is a survivor. If the right combination of anti-TB drugs is not used or if they are not taken long enough, the bacteria can change and become resistant to treatment. Incorrect or incomplete treatment gives TB bacteria a chance to become immune to the drugs that can kill them. As the bacteria adapt to the treatment, the best anti-TB antibiotics become less effective against them and a tougher strain of TB, called multidrug-resistant TB, develops. If TB becomes resistant to the best anti-TB drugs, alternative drugs can be used to treat it but they are less effective, more toxic, more expensive, and the outcomes of treatment are often worse. Global rates of multidrug-resistant TB have been tracked since the late 1990s.

Extensively drug-resistant TB is a relatively rare but deadly type of multidrug-resistant TB that is unaffected by almost all anti-TB drugs. This highly resistant form of TB has been identified in every region of the world, including the United States. Treatment-resistant TB is a significant problem in poor and developing countries because people who are sick with the disease may not have access to complete medical care for a long enough period of time, which gives the bacteria an opportunity to become immune to treatment. Multidrug-resistant TB is a common problem in places like Africa, Haiti, Russia, and China, and it greatly intensifies the current global burden of TB.

TB can be cured with the right treatment regimen, but if TB or multidrug-resistant TB is left untreated, it may be fatal. TB unfolds as a progression from exposure to infection to disease. The advance of TB from one step to the next varies from person to person, and depending on individual and environmental circumstances, it may either stop at any point or continue to become increasingly more serious.

Multidrug-Resistant TB in the Former Soviet States

According to data gathered from more than 90,000 patients in 83 countries between 2002 and 2007, the countries of the former Soviet Union reported the highest rates of multidrug-resistant TB in the world. In some former Soviet states and cities during these years, the percentage of cases that were resistant to the first-line anti-TB drugs was between 7 percent and 22 percent, including 19 percent of cases in Moldova and 22 percent of cases in the city of Baku, Azerbaijan (Wright, 2009).

FROM EXPOSURE TO INFECTION

When a person who is infected with pulmonary TB coughs, sneezes, or speaks, droplets containing disease-producing bacteria are propelled out into the air. Many tiny droplets containing the germ become airborne with every cough or sneeze from an infected person. The droplets dry quickly in the air, where they can float around for several hours waiting to be inhaled by another person. Once contagious droplets are inhaled, the person is now exposed to TB. Depending on the circumstance, the newly exposed person may or may not go on to develop TB infection or disease. The body is equipped with defense mechanisms to protect it and when the germ is inhaled, most of the larger droplets become trapped in the nose and throat, and infection does not usually develop. Even though a small number of infectious microorganisms may get beyond this initial line of defense and reach the lungs, the lungs are also equipped to fight TB. If the defenses in the lungs also fail, exposure to the germ that causes TB may result in infection.

The chance of developing TB infection after exposure to the bacteria is much more likely when certain environmental and personal risk factors are present. For example, overcrowded living conditions (such as those that exist in prisons or nursing homes), close contact with someone who has already has TB, poor nutrition, urban living, homelessness, intravenous (I.V.) drug use, alcoholism, and human immunodeficiency virus/acquired immunodeficiency syndrome (HIV/AIDS) all increase the risk that exposure to TB will result in a progression to infection.

FROM INFECTION TO DISEASE

Just as exposure to TB does not always lead to infection, TB infection does not always lead to full-blown TB disease. Throughout the world, more than two billion people are currently infected with TB, but of this number only about 10 percent will go on to develop TB disease. If disease occurs, most of the time it happens during the first one or two years following infection. Even when a person is infected with TB, a strong immune system can still successfully fight it.

When the immune system initially wins the battle with M. *tuberculosis*, bacteria can remain alive in the body for many years without doing any harm. TB that is present in the body in an inactive state is called latent TB. This type of TB is not infectious, it causes no symptoms, and the person who has it is not sick. However, if the immune system at some point becomes weakened by factors such as other diseases or old age, the latent bacteria, like tiny time bombs, may reactivate and produce active TB infection. If latent TB is discovered, it may be treated with antibiotic drugs to prevent active disease from developing in the future. Whether latent TB is treated often depends on the patient's individual risk factors for developing active TB at a later date. For example, patients with HIV and latent TB are advised to be treated with anti-TB drugs. Since latent TB produces fewer bacteria than active infection, treatment is usually easier and can be accomplished with just one antibiotic instead of the usual combination of antibiotics that is required to treat full-blown TB.

The risk of developing active TB disease either immediately following infection (primary TB) or later on if latent bacteria reactivate (secondary TB) is mostly related to specific factors that are associated with the person who is infected. For example, age is an important determinant of how the TB infection will progress. Among infected people, the incidence of TB disease is highest in adolescents and young adults. Risk of disease may also increase for elderly people, possibly because the immune system is weakened by age or the presence of other diseases. The strength of the particular M. *tuberculosis* bacteria that caused the infection, whether there has been prior or extensive exposure to TB, and the health of the immune system are additional factors that influence whether TB infection will progress to disease or become latent.

Because HIV/AIDS suppresses immune function, it is the most prominent risk factor associated with progression from latent TB infection to active TB disease. In the world today, HIV is the only infectious disease that is more deadly than TB and because HIV/AIDS impairs immune response, people who are infected with it are at very high risk of also developing TB. Because of this deadly one-two punch, the worldwide prevalence of AIDS and HIV is a major challenge in controlling the spread of TB. A significant percentage of people infected with HIV also have TB, and people infected with both diseases are at a greater risk of complications and death than those who are infected with either disease alone. The lethal relationship that exists between these two deadly infectious diseases greatly contributes to the current global burden of TB.

THE DEVELOPMENT OF DISEASE

Similar to the different ways that TB bacteria behaves once it comes in contact with a potential new victim—either having no effect, causing active infection, or being present but latent—TB disease also travels diverse paths. While some untreated people develop severe pulmonary TB within a few weeks or months after the onset of the disease and others experience spontaneous remission, most begin a chronic, progressively debilitating disease course.

The first contact between TB bacteria and its human host occurs when air containing droplets of bacteria is inhaled and some droplets reach the small air sacs in the lungs called alveoli; this is where TB infection may begin. In a healthy person, the immune system is called to attention and it responds to the invading bacteria. Powerful white blood cells called macrophages are called forth to move in and swallow the TB bacteria. Macrophages surround and engulf the bacteria but, at this point, the cells are immature and have not been activated by additional help from the immune system to enable them to destroy the bacteria.

The powerless macrophages now contain multiplying bacteria and they begin to mass together inside the alveoli. Other white blood cells, such as T cells, respond to the bacterial invasion and join the cluster of accumulating macrophages. Within several weeks, this collection of cells forms a hard, gray, swelling lesion called a tubercle. In the majority of people, a strong immune response now occurs to stop the disease process. The T cells produce chemicals that activate the macrophages and signal them to kill the TB bacteria or stop them from growing. While these immune reactions help stop the invading bacteria, the protective response also causes damage to some lung cells.

As the immune response continues, the tubercle may still grow larger and destroy surrounding lung tissue. Cells begin to die inside the tubercle and a soft, semi-solid material that resembles soft cheese, called caseous necrosis, is produced. Around the outside of the tubercle, a tough scar tissue forms to trap the germs inside. The trapped bacteria can remain alive inside the acidic and oxygen-deprived environment of the tubercle for an extended period of time, but they cannot multiply. As the immune system takes control of the infection, the tubercles heal and become scarred and calcified. It is through this healing process that the TB infection becomes latent.

However, if the immune response is weak, such as in people with HIV, it cannot contain the bacteria and make them inactive. The bacteria multiply, burst out of the tubercle, and continue to reproduce in the surrounding lung tissue. More lung tissue is replaced by caseous necrosis, which may gradually turn to liquid. *M. tuberculosis* grows very well in this liquid environment and rapid reproduction of the bacteria occurs. The liquid leftovers from dead cells and bacteria are carried up the airway by mucus flow in the lungs, leaving behind cavities and scar tissue. The mucus irritates the lungs and coughing, one of the first signs of TB, begins. Eventually, the bacteria may break through the walls of the alveoli and enter the tiny blood vessels that surround the air sacs, causing blood to appear in the material that is brought up from the lungs with a cough. The material that is discharged from the air passages during coughing is called sputum. It contains mucus and other byproducts of the infection, including bacteria. As more lung tissue is damaged, fewer working alveoli are left. Without working lung tissue, the exchange of oxygen is compromised, cells cannot work properly, and symptoms appear throughout the body. Breathing becomes more difficult, the infected person feels tired, and weight loss begins. If left untreated, TB can progress very quickly but it usually becomes a long-term and chronic disease during which the patient becomes progressively more ill.

DISCOVERING THE CAUSE: THE GERM THEORY OF DISEASE

M. *Tuberculosis* has been around since ancient times. Although the biology of TB is very well understood now, many centuries passed during which the cause of TB remained a mystery. For a very long time, it was believed that certain people had a hereditary predisposition to developing TB. In a way, this made as much sense as anything else since multiple cases of TB within one family were a common occurrence. However, speculation and suspicion relating to the outlandish idea that living creatures, invisible to the naked eye, might be responsible for the transmission of TB from one person to another buzzed around the outskirts of mainstream medicine for many years. But as late as the 19th century, conjecture about contagion as the cause of TB did not stand up to the statistical facts, the knowledge of pathology, or the reasoning of the day, and a germ theory of disease was routinely rejected by conventional medical authorities.

Acceptance of the reality that TB was caused by microorganisms would require more than the imagination and guesswork of forward thinking scientists and physicians—extensive scientific experimentation and proof were needed to change the course of medical history. Scientific proof requires the use of strict criteria to minimize the chance that personal or cultural bias will creep in and influence how findings are interpreted. Scientists and doctors began to unravel the cause of TB by observing the disease, using educated guesses to explain what they saw and might expect to see, and performing experiments to see if their ideas were right. Rigorous scientific method allowed them to prove the germ theory of disease and to discover the cause of TB.

Toward that end, French military surgeon Jean Antoine Villemin (1827–1892) made great strides by demonstrating that phthisis, as TB was known in those days, could be transmitted from one animal to another. From experience with horses in his youth, Villemin was familiar with a horse disease that could be transmitted to people. This disease as it occurred in humans reminded Villemin of TB and in March 1865, he began pioneering laboratory experiments on animals to discover more about TB.

In an attempt to reproduce TB in healthy animals, Villemin harvested tuberculous material from the lung cavity of a patient who had just died of TB and placed a small amount of it into the bodies of two rabbits through small incisions he made in the skin. Two other rabbits were inoculated in a similar manner, but instead of using tuberculous matter he placed tissue fluid from a burn blister into the incisions. The experiment was set—the two animals that had been exposed to TB could be compared to the two animals that had only been exposed to material from a burn. Two months later, the animals were killed so that Villemin could examine the effects the different exposures had produced. Villemin found what he was looking for—in the two animals that had been inoculated with tuberculous material, Villemin found widespread pulmonary and lymph node TB; in the other two animals, there was no evidence of TB. But even though scientific evidence pointing to the existence of germs was beginning to displace speculation, most of the medical authorities of the day were not yet ready to believe it.

In contrast to most scientific research of the time, Villemin's experiments were performed with extraordinary care, and the procedures and results were well documented. All together, he conducted six series of experiments using tuberculous material from humans and six more using tuberculous material taken from the udder of an infected cow. The results from every experiment were consistent—the animals exposed to tuberculous matter got TB while the others did not. Villemin was convinced that TB was a specific infection that was transmitted by something that was present in dead tuberculous material. Two years after he began his experiments, he was ready to present his discoveries to the preeminent medical authority in France, the Académie de Médecine. The Académie was a traditional place, deeply steeped in the theory that TB was the result of specific family-related characteristics. Despite Villemin's scientific rigor and the compelling results of his experiments, the Académie refused to publish his work. Not one to be dismissed so lightly, Villemin proceeded to publish his findings on his own, but his colleagues followed the thinking of the Académie and his inspired work never received much recognition in France. Beyond the valuable insight that Villemin gained into the nature of TB, his experiments also taught him that challenging tradition to advance a new way of thinking is not an easy prospect.

Villemin's body of work in TB was advanced by Louis Pasteur (1822–1895), a French scientist and microbiologist who is best known for discoveries that helped to elucidate the causes and prevention of disease. His work is intertwined with the history of TB in a variety of ways. As a professor of chemistry, he demonstrated that fermentation was caused by the growth of microorganisms. His experiments helped to develop and support the germ theory by showing that under laboratory conditions microorganisms did not spontaneously generate from nonliving matter. His study of fermentation and microbes became the basis of the technique that is used kill bacteria in milk. Named in honor of Pasteur, pasteurization is the process whereby milk is heated to between 60 and 80 degrees centigrade for about 20 minutes and then rapidly cooled. Pasteurization was widely used to help clean up the diary industry and control the milk-borne spread of bovine TB.

The Consequences of Questioning Traditional TB Authority

In the 1840s, an unconventional country doctor in England named George Boding-ton (1811–1882) also suffered the intellectual consequences of challenging TB. In an essay that was critical of standard medical treatment given to patients with TB, Bodington expressed his contrary opinions in a manner that was considered by his peers to be both disrespectful and arrogant. His vehemence and tone were so inflammatory that he enraged his colleagues and became something of a medical outcast. He attacked the current drugs that were used for TB patients, criticized the practice of putting patients in closed-up rooms, and condemned doctors who cured TB patients by sending them to temperate climates where they would frequently die anyway.

His positive recommendations for treatment—fresh air, short walks, and a nutritious diet—were considered to be just as unorthodox as his criticism, and he was thoroughly maligned when he opened a small facility to treat patients who desired his regimen. Letters from the most esteemed doctors of the day poured into the prestigious medical journal *The Lancet* expressing the opinion that Bodington's "very crude" ideas were best left to fall into a "well-merited oblivion." Bodington's practice slowly dwindled, and his personal life subsequently became very unstable. In the late 1850s, Bodington went insane and was sent to live in an asylum. By the time he died, in 1882, medical discoveries had begun to illuminate the nature of TB and Bodington's formerly eccentric opinions no longer seemed quite so far-fetched. Upon his death, *The Lancet* once again offered commentary, this time with a note of surprise that "a simple country doctor...should have arrived at conclusions which anticipated some of our most recent teachings. It is alas less surprising that he met the usual fate of those who question authority." The final words of recognition from *The Lancet* were too little and too late for Dr. Bodington.

In his later years of work on disease prevention, Pasteur experimented with the use of artificially weakened disease organisms to induce immunity in animals. This greatly advanced the development of vaccines, and Pasteur was the first to produce a vaccine against rabies by growing the virus in rabbits and then weakening it. The vaccine was used on a boy who had been badly bitten by a rabid dog and it was an unqualified success. Although Pasteur was not the first scientist to advance a germ theory, his groundbreaking work served as the next plateau of knowledge and inspired the important developments that were yet to come.

The next advancement in the proof of a germ theory of disease forever changed the trajectory of TB and formed the basis of the first real step toward a cure. Twenty years after Villemin and his work had fallen into obscurity, new discoveries by a German scientist named Robert Koch (1843–1910) proved the germ theory of TB contagion and he, not Villemin, rose to international acclaim. Koch was a microbiologist whose first research interest involved anthrax, another savage disease that took its toll on animals and sometimes on humans. He conducted exacting experiments and proved that anthrax was caused by a specific and identifiable type of bacteria. Additionally, he showed that anthrax bacteria could lie dormant in certain circumstances but could later revive, start reproducing, and kill again when they were transferred to a new living host.

Using his work with anthrax as a foundation to build on, Koch performed his first experiments with TB when he harvested specimens containing TB from the body of a young man who had died of the disease within a few short weeks of experiencing his first symptoms. Koch started by injecting the samples from the dead patient into guinea pigs and rabbits. Using a special technique that he developed to grow and stain the bacteria, he began looking for the culprit that caused TB. To be sure that he was identifying the actual causative organism, Koch imposed three strict criteria on the way he conducted his TB experiments and interpreted the results. To prove that any organism he found was the real cause of TB, Koch reasoned that it must be found in every tubercular lesion he

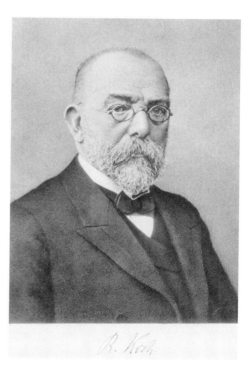

Robert Koch, the pioneering microbiologist who discovered the bacteria that cause TB. Courtesy of the National Library of Medicine.

examined, it must be capable of being reproduced for several generations outside the human body in the laboratory, and in the end, it must be able to cause the original illness in laboratory animals all over again.

Like others before him who had looked for the bacterial cause of TB, at first Koch was not able to see anything under the microscope because M. *tuberculosis* does not easily stain with dyes. Finally, Koch had some luck coloring the bacteria using an old dye preparation and through a bit of imaginative detective work, he figured out why. The dye had successfully colored the TB organisms because it had been contaminated with some ammonia that was present in the air of the laboratory. This chance discovery became the basis for the regular use of specific chemical compounds to enhance the staining process of M. *tuberculosis*. In an additional moment of serendipity, a stained tissue sample that had been prepared on a slide was inadvertently left on the hot surface of a stove. When the neglected slide was examined the next day, the bacilli were found to be brilliantly stained; from then on, heating became an integral part of the staining process for M. *tuberculosis*. It wasn't long before Koch's investigations and methods paid off. In a matter of just a few months, he was able to observe the rod-shaped organisms that he suspected were the cause of TB. For the first time, M. *tuberculosis* was observed and identified, marking a turning point in the history of a disease that had held humans hostage since the beginning of time.

In those days, the practice of medicine was mostly based on practical skills and common sense experience. Science was not held in particularly high esteem, and Koch's approach to finding the cause of TB was seen as rigid and contrary to the traditional healing approach used by the leaders in the field. In spite of resistance from his peers, after Koch discovered M. *tuberculosis* bacteria, he persevered and managed to satisfy all his predetermined criteria of success. Because of their shape and cellular composition, the bacteria that cause TB were (and remain today) a very difficult organism to culture. By using his inventive and meticulous methods, Koch was able to prove that M. *tuberculosis* existed and was responsible for the transmission of TB. In what can only be called an indisputable scientific triumph, all that remained was convincing the world that he was right.

In 1882, Koch presented his irrefutable evidence of the existence of M. *tuberculosis* to a prestigious medical meeting in Berlin, Germany. He clearly described his evidence to prove that TB was caused by a specific microorganism, and he explained the special techniques that were needed to stain and culture them. Although news of the discovery of the microorganism that caused TB traveled quickly and hopefully throughout the world, the existence of M. *tuberculosis* was also initially greeted with resistance and skepticism in traditional medical circles. It wasn't long, however, before other scientists began to replicate Koch's findings in their laboratories and doubts about the authenticity of the germ theory of TB became more difficult to sustain. With each new piece of supportive evidence, it became increasingly apparent that the skeptics whose beliefs were based on tradition and stubbornness were losing ground to the facts produced by science.

New Yorkers wasted no time in reacting to the news that an infectious cause of TB had been discovered. In New York City, at Bellevue Hospital, the practice of sputum examination for all patients suspected of having TB was instituted and the results were used as the basis for a conclusive diagnosis of the disease. One initial nonbeliever in the germ theory became a convert when he demonstrated that TB bacteria in infected sputum could be ground underneath a shoe, dried, moistened, dried again, and remoistened eight more times, after which it could still kill a guinea pig. In 1886, France enacted the first legislation prohibiting spitting in public places and in 1887, a hospital in London instituted the practice of emptying and disinfecting the spittoons used by TB patients.

In 1889, a report issued by the New York City Health Department set forth the concepts of TB and suggested measures for preventing its spread. In light of Koch's discovery, it declared that TB was not an inherited condition but a "distinctly preventable" disease that was acquired by direct transmission of TB bacteria from the sick to the healthy. To prevent the spread of disease, official inspection of cattle, public education to inform people with TB they were an "actual source of danger" to others, and careful disinfection of hospital rooms were among the recommended actions. Although most physicians did not believe that official measures were needed, these health department edicts marked the beginning of what would become an active and sometimes invasive public health campaign to prevent and control TB.

The world welcomed Koch's discovery of M. *tuberculosis*, an advance that would eventually lead to a cure for TB. With the knowledge that TB was caused by a microorganism, the science of microbiology was born. Calling TB by names from the past—phthisis, consumption, the King's Evil, the wasting illness—was no longer suitable now that the cause of the disease was known. In 1839,

---

M. *Tuberculosis* Gets the Nobel Prize

The Nobel Prize was first awarded in 1901 and quickly became the most prestigious award in the world of medicine. Robert Koch was disappointed that he was not the recipient of the Prize during the first few years that it was presented, but his work in the field of TB and his discovery of the cause of the dreaded disease were eventually acknowledged when he was awarded the Nobel Prize in 1905.

"tuberculosis" had been suggested for use as a generic term to describe all forms of phthisis because the tubercle was the fundamental basis of all forms of the disease. After Koch's discovery, the word *tuberculosis* evolved to refer to any disease that was caused by tubercle bacilli, whether or not lesions were found in the infected organ. When the perception of TB shifted from an anatomical perspective to a bacteriological position, a new understanding of the disease that had plagued generations was born.

2

Signs and Certainty: Tuberculosis Symptoms and Diagnosis

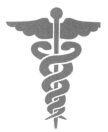

T
he key to diagnosing TB begins with a high degree of suspicion that the disease may be present. TB should be suspected if suggestive physical symptoms and high-risk factors, such as a crowded living environment, prison, HIV infection, or immigration from a place with high TB incidence, are present. Ultimately, TB can only be diagnosed when M. *tuberculosis* bacteria are identified in a specimen, like sputum, that comes from the patient. While other laboratory and clinical findings may strongly suggest a diagnosis of TB, they cannot confirm it. Symptoms of TB along with suspect environmental or individual factors should quickly prompt the diagnostic process to begin.

SYMPTOMS

If physical symptoms suggest the presence of TB, a complete evaluation of the patient is required. Personal information about the person's country of origin, age, and ethnic or racial group can help doctors identify people who may be at increased risk of infection. A comprehensive medical history including information about prior TB exposure, infection, or disease, and the presence of other medical conditions, such as HIV, helps determine if TB infection is

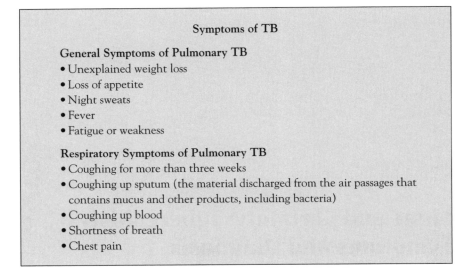

Symptoms of TB

General Symptoms of Pulmonary TB
- Unexplained weight loss
- Loss of appetite
- Night sweats
- Fever
- Fatigue or weakness

Respiratory Symptoms of Pulmonary TB
- Coughing for more than three weeks
- Coughing up sputum (the material discharged from the air passages that contains mucus and other products, including bacteria)
- Coughing up blood
- Shortness of breath
- Chest pain

probable. Physical examination provides additional knowledge about a patient's overall condition. Symptoms of TB that occur in less obvious circumstances, such as persistent coughing by a student living in a college dorm, may not prompt high suspicion among health care workers and a TB diagnosis may be easily missed.

It may be many months from the time of exposure to TB bacteria until the physical symptoms of the infection develop. In the medical world, TB is known as a great pretender because of its varied symptom presentations. However, general physical symptoms do help identify active TB disease, and if TB is in the lungs, symptoms specific to the respiratory system are also easily identifiable. If TB is active in a part of the body other than the lungs (extra-pulmonary TB), the symptoms of infection will depend on what part of the body is involved.

THE TOOLS OF DIAGNOSIS

In poor countries, it is estimated that fewer than half of patients are correctly diagnosed with TB the first time they seek help. Delayed TB diagnosis is related to several bad outcomes including increased patient suffering, greater likelihood of infecting someone else, higher costs to the patient due to factors such as more time lost from work, and less successful treatment of patients who have both TB and HIV. Factors that contribute to delayed diagnosis include the severity of the disease, lack of access to health care services, poverty, gender, inadequate expertise of medical personnel, and failure to seek treatment promptly because of the stigma attached to TB.

Even though TB remains one of the leading causes of death worldwide from infectious disease, diagnostic methods are still rather limited. In low-income countries where health care resources are scarce, case finding and diagnosis often still rely on a physician's ability to recognize the symptoms of TB. Several laboratory tests and clinical tools are available to help diagnose TB, but only a handful of tests are considered diagnostically certain.

Tuberculin Skin Test

The Mantoux test is the skin test that is used as a diagnostic tool for TB in the United States. A small amount of tuberculin, a sterile solution containing substances extracted from dead tuberculosis bacteria, is injected just beneath the skin on the forearm. A positive reaction to a skin test does not mean that there is active M. *tuberculosis* in the body; rather, a positive response means that a person has developed an immune response to the bacteria that cause TB, indicating that they have been exposed to TB at some point.

If a person has been exposed to TB bacteria, within 48 to 72 hours an immune response develops in reaction to the injection and a hardened, red swelling occurs at the injection site. The reaction must be interpreted carefully and the test result is considered positive for TB only in relation to a person's medical risk factors. For example, a smaller swelling (between five and ten millimeters) is considered a positive skin test result for someone with HIV infection or recent contact with a TB patient; for someone with no known TB risk factors, only a larger area of swelling (bigger than 10 millimeters) is considered a positive skin test result. A positive skin test reaction alone is not enough to establish a TB diagnosis because it does not distinguish between latent and active TB infection. Additionally, since an immune response does not occur for several weeks after infection, a TB skin test given too soon after infection occurs may be falsely negative. A false negative skin test result can also occur in people who have diseases that weaken the immune system, like AIDS or cancer.

In most developing countries, a vaccine called the Bacillus Calmette-Guérin (BCG) is given to babies at birth to reduce the most severe consequences of TB in infants and children. Individuals who have been vaccinated with BCG will have a positive reaction to a skin test since they have produced an immune response to TB from the vaccination. The vaccine is not used in the United States and its effectiveness for preventing TB in adults is questionable. Since a person who has been vaccinated with BCG may subsequently have a positive reaction to a TB skin test, this makes detecting TB later in their life much more difficult.

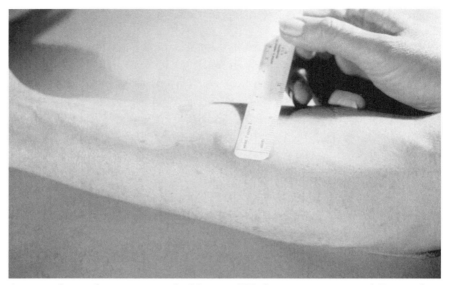

A patient having his reaction to the Mantoux TB skin test site measured. During the skin test, fluid called tuberculin is injected under the skin of the forearm. If a patient is infected with TB, 24–48 hours after the test the injection site becomes hard, swollen, and red. Courtesy of the Centers for Disease Control and Prevention.

Skin tests are not used as a general screening tool for TB, but they are used to help identify TB in individuals who are at high risk of having the disease. People with signs, symptoms, and/or laboratory abnormalities suggestive of active TB are likely to be given a TB skin test. People who are poor, elderly, medically underserved, homeless, HIV or AIDS positive, prison inmates, alcoholic, or I.V. drug users are also at high risk for TB infection and are good candidates for skin-test screening. In some countries, individuals who are emigrating from countries with high rates of TB incidence may be screened for TB with skin tests. Health care or other workers (e.g., prison guards) who come in contact with high-risk populations may be screened in relation to their employment. In addition, a TB skin test may also be done as part of a physical examination prior to starting school or a new job. When someone has a positive reaction to a TB skin test, additional tests are required to confirm or rule out a diagnosis of TB.

Tuberculosis Blood Testing

A blood test called the QuantiFERON®-TB Gold (QFT-G) is another method used to help diagnose TB infection. Unlike a TB skin test, QFT-G results are not affected by prior BCG vaccination. Approved for use in the United States in 2005, the QFT-G measures the immune response to TB proteins when they are mixed with a small amount of blood. A positive result suggests that M. *tuberculosis* is present, while a negative result indicates that infection is unlikely. Latent TB can also be diagnosed by the QFT-G test, but a medical evaluation must rule out the presence of active TB first. The QFT-G blood test can be used in all situations where a skin test is appropriate and results can be available within 24 hours. When someone has a positive reaction to a TB skin test or the QFT-G blood test, additional tests are performed to confirm or rule out a diagnosis of TB.

Chest X-Ray

An abnormal chest x-ray may be suggestive of TB, but it can never be considered fully diagnostic. The purpose of a chest x-ray is to check for lung abnormalities in people who have symptoms of pulmonary TB disease, or to rule out the possibility of TB in a person who has a positive skin test reaction and no symptoms of disease. Usually, when a person has pulmonary TB disease, the chest x-ray

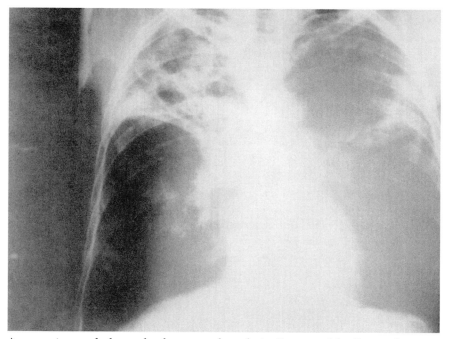

An x-ray image of advanced pulmonary tuberculosis. Courtesy of the Centers for Disease Control and Prevention.

appears abnormal. For example, collections of fluid and cells, cavities, and lesions of differing size, shape, and density may be seen on an x-ray of a person who has TB currently or who has had TB in the past. However, like positive TB skin or blood test, an x-ray alone cannot be used to make a definitive TB diagnosis.

Smear and Culture Testing

A definitive diagnosis of tuberculosis can only be made by finding M. *tuberculosis* organisms in a specimen (usually sputum produced by coughing) obtained from a patient. To help identify what microorganisms are present in a specimen, bacteria are stained in the laboratory using a technique that dyes tissues and germs so that they can be viewed more easily under a microscope. Mycobacteria, the kind of bacteria that causes TB, are characteristically impermeable to dye when they are stained. However, when stained mycobacteria are heated and treated with acidified organic compounds, the dye is retained and the colored organisms become visible under the microscope. Bacteria, such as mycobacteria, that react to staining in this way are called acid-fast bacteria.

In a laboratory test called a smear, the specimen provided by the patient is examined for the presence of acid-fast M. *tuberculosis*. A specifically prepared glass slide is spread with the sputum sample, treated with special stain, and examined under a microscope. Since M. *tuberculosis* is the most commonly encountered acid-fast bacteria, finding acid-fast microorganisms on a smear highly suggests a diagnosis of TB.

To absolutely determine if the acid-fast bacteria detected on the smear are M. *tuberculosis*, the sputum sample is also incubated and the bacteria are allowed to grow during a test called a culture. Acid-fast bacteria cultures are performed on respiratory samples that are decontaminated of normal respiratory bacteria and concentrated to increase the ability to detect mycobacteria. Nutrients and incubation provide a friendly environment for the slow growing mycobacteria. The result of a culture is definitive. The exact type of bacteria and the drugs that are likely to kill them can both be identified once the bacteria are cultured. The growth and detection of M. *tuberculosis* in a culture requires up to eight weeks; cultures are held for six to eight weeks before they are reported as negative for M. *tuberculosis*. A positive culture for M. *tuberculosis* finally confirms the diagnosis of TB.

Nucleic Acid Amplification Tests

Direct molecular methods to identify M. *tuberculosis* do not require the growth of the bacteria. A genetic probe or molecular TB test provides diagnostic

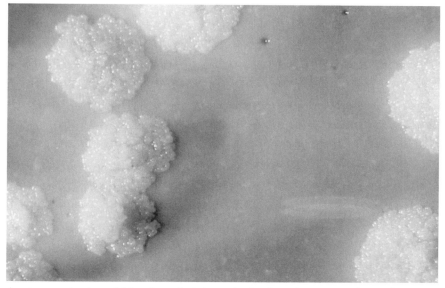

A microscopic view of M. *tuberculosis* bacteria that have been grown in a culture.
It shows how the bacteria cluster closely together in a colony and the typical colorless
rough surface structure. Courtesy of the Centers for Disease Control and Prevention.

information by amplifying or replicating the genetic components of the bacteria. Tests of this nature have been available for more than a decade, but they have not been frequently used in the United States. Nucleic acid amplification (NAA) tests identify the presence of genetic information unique to M. *tuberculosis* in preprocessed respiratory samples. The NAA technique uses chemical rather than biological ways to form extra copies of M. *tuberculosis* genes in the sample so that they are present at levels that can be reliably detected within 24 to 48 hours. Earlier laboratory confirmation of TB can lead to the quicker start of treatment, improved outcomes for the patient, and a better chance of stopping transmission of the disease to other people. Recommendations made by the Centers for Disease Control in January 2009 state that NAA should be performed on at least one respiratory sample taken from every patient with signs and symptoms of pulmonary TB who does not have a confirmed TB diagnosis and for whom the test results would change the way the case is managed or the way TB control is performed. Because of the high cost of molecular genetic methods of detection and the need for highly equipped laboratories to perform the tests, TB diagnosis still relies heavily on the use of sputum smear and culture tests.

Is It Tuberculosis Infection or Disease?

Infection
- M. *tuberculosis* is present
- TB skin test is positive
- Chest x-ray is normal
- Sputum smears and cultures are negative
- There are no symptoms
- The person is not infectious
- This is not defined as a case of TB

Disease
- M. *tuberculosis* is present
- TB skin test is positive
- Chest x-ray may show lesions
- Sputum smears and cultures are positive
- Symptoms (e.g., cough, fever) are present
- The person is infectious
- This is defined as a case of TB

DIAGNOSIS IN DEVELOPING COUNTRIES

The current TB crisis is having a much greater impact on people in developing nations of the world than it is on people in more affluent nations. Although great advances have been made in improving treatment regimens and increasing patient access to health care in developing countries, the diagnosis of TB remains a stumbling block in the effort to improve services in the countries that bear the highest TB burden. Since the global strategy for controlling TB depends on treating the sick and interrupting transmission of new cases, improving the ability to detect TB is critical. If TB remains undiagnosed and untreated, symptoms become worse and the disease progresses; young people, malnourished people, and people who have compromised immune systems are especially susceptible to rapid progressions of disease.

Currently, examining a sputum specimen under a microscope for the presence of TB bacteria is the only diagnostic test that is available to most people in the world where TB is a major health problem. This is essentially the same method of identifying bacteria that was used by Robert Koch when he discovered the bacteria in the latter part of the 19th century, and in the developing world, sputum microscopy has severe limitations. For example, diagnostic accuracy in HIV-positive individuals is poor, cultural sensitivities may interfere with the ability to obtain a sputum sample, and it usually takes several weeks to obtain results. Delayed diagnosis may result in considerable loss of income, substantial travel costs for patients who live in rural locations, longer periods of infectiousness, and delayed start of treatment.

In light of the escalating incidence of multidrug-resistant TB, it is of additional concern that people who seek treatment in developing countries are usually not tested for drug sensitivity because the availability of resources to do so is limited. If someone is infected with a strain of TB that is resistant to first-line anti-TB drugs and health care providers are unaware, it is likely that an incorrect treatment regimen will be prescribed. When the means to test for drug susceptibility are not available, a patient with a drug-resistant strain of TB may remain vulnerable to persistent illness and continued infectiousness.

The costs associated with diagnosis substantially increase the challenge of detecting TB in developing countries. Because the highest burden of TB is found in poor countries and prevalence of the disease is higher among poor people, it is important to understand the factors associated with the cost of being diagnosed with TB. For example, in an urban area of the African country of Malawi, the cost of receiving a TB diagnosis is prohibitively high for patients and households, even though basic health care services are provided free. Beyond medical intervention, the cost of a TB diagnosis includes indirect factors like transportation, food, and the value of lost income. In Malawi, the total cost of diagnosis is higher for poor patients than for patients who are not poor, and the costs are also greater for poor households or when the person with TB is a woman. To improve TB diagnosis among the poor in developing countries, cost-effective diagnostic strategies must be identified and used.

Organizations are stepping up to the challenge of improving TB diagnostics in developing nations. On the eve of World TB Day 2001 (held annually on March 24) the Bill & Melinda Gates Foundation awarded $10 million to a special program at the World Health Organization to facilitate the development of new tests for the diagnosis of TB. The five-year grant supporting the Tuberculosis Diagnostic Initiative helped to speed up research efforts to develop new approaches for detecting TB among patients with symptoms of the disease. Work is also under way to find simple and accurate methods to quickly detect bacterial resistance to treatment and to uncover latent infection or developing disease in persons without symptoms. In developing nations, simple TB tests and diagnostic methods that can be brought to a patient in any location, no matter how remote, are needed as well. The Foundation for Innovative New Diagnostics is another TB control initiative that is coordinating the work of nearly 40 companies,

---

Cultural Differences Matter

In some countries, such as Pakistan and Bangladesh, women are not allowed to spit. Producing a sputum sample to test for the presence of M. *tuberculosis* bacteria may be a culturally sensitive issue for some patients in developing countries.

academic institutions, and government bodies to develop TB tests that can be used wherever they are needed and are easy, inexpensive, and accurate.

TUBERCULOSIS IN SUBGROUPS OF PEOPLE

TB does not occur at the same rates or for the same reasons in all groups of people. Prison inmates (see chapter 7), people who abuse alcohol, I.V. drug users, immigrants, the elderly, and people with HIV/AIDS (see chapter 7) are among the groups of people who are more likely to get TB. Social conditions, the strength of the immune response, and biological differences contribute to higher rates of TB among different groups of people.

Women

Given that key symptoms are associated with TB, it is not surprising that the World Health Organization advocates that diagnostics be performed in all patients from countries with high TB prevalence who cough for longer than three weeks and cough up blood. In settings with widespread poverty and limited medical resources, detecting cases of TB mostly relies on the ability of the health care provider to recognize patients with these symptoms. Worldwide, TB is the greatest single infectious cause of death in young women. While fewer women than men are diagnosed with TB, a greater percentage of female TB patients die of it. Since it has been suggested that woman with TB are often diagnosed later than men, diagnosis on the basis of only key symptoms may present some difficulties for female patients.

The symptoms of TB may present differently in women than in men. For example, it is believed that women with TB may cough up blood less frequently than men, and some evidence shows that extra-pulmonary TB may be more common in women than men. Additionally, biological differences may exist between men and women in regard to pulmonary lesions; for example, the area of the lung where lesions are typically located may not be the same for women as it is for men. Differences such as these may have an effect on the sensitivity of sputum testing used to diagnose TB.

Up to 70 percent of deaths due to TB in women occur during the childbearing years, but information on TB diagnosis and treatment in pregnant women is limited (World Health Organization, 2001). How TB affects the health of the mother-to-be, the fetus, and the newborn infant is not fully understood and information about the effects of anti-TB drugs during pregnancy is inadequate. Women commonly believe that pregnancy makes it more difficult to tolerate TB drugs or that it makes the drugs ineffective, which may lead them to interrupt TB treatment when they become pregnant. Stopping treatment before TB is cured leaves a woman vulnerable to relapse and the development of multidrug resistance. The lack of information regarding TB and pregnancy means that there are no available guidelines to help health care professionals diagnose and manage pregnant patients with TB, and there is little information available to help a woman take care of herself and her baby.

Cultural differences may also account for some disparities among women and men in relation to the experience of TB. In some developing countries, it has been shown that women are more likely to be concerned about the social stigma of TB, whereas men are more concerned about the economic impact of the disease. In traditional male-dominated societies, the stigma and consequences associated with having TB may be much greater for women than for men. Potential consequences for a woman diagnosed with TB include ostracism by the community, abandonment by her husband and/or his family, divorce or the addition of a second wife to the family, loss of social and economic support, loss of housing, or denial of access to her children. Marriage chances may be diminished for a woman who is known to have TB or to have a family member with TB since the stigma associated with the disease may affect all members of a household. As a result, some families go to great lengths to deny or hide an unmarried daughter's illness.

Additionally, since traditional women's roles are usually related to more activities inside the house, women and men may be predisposed to different risk factors for exposure. Men are commonly exposed to TB in social settings, whereas women may be more vulnerable to TB exposure when taking care of sick family members, doing household chores, and engaging in intimate and prolonged contact with members of the extended family. For a variety of gender-based and cultural reasons, women and men may experience different effects and consequences of TB. Given the biology of the disease and the societies in which it occurs, the expected standards of TB may in actuality be the male standards of TB. Unique factors may influence a woman's vulnerability to exposure, the way her symptoms may become apparent, and the way she seeks care once she realizes she is sick.

Children

Young children have high rates of TB in both developing countries around the globe and in the poorest communities in highly developed nations. In developing countries where a large proportion of the population is under 15 years of age, as many as 40 percent of TB cases may occur in children. Active pulmonary TB is the most common source of TB infection in children and they are most frequently exposed to it through contact with infectious adults. As long as infectious adults remain untreated, children will continue to be at risk for TB. In addition, TB is difficult to diagnose in children. Even where laboratory facilities are good, confirming the presence of TB through sputum culture is not easy to do in children. Many children in developing countries are vaccinated against TB at birth, and although vaccination protects infants from the devastation of TB, it is not believed to prevent active TB in adulthood. Vaccination has never been a part of TB control efforts in the United States. Curing TB in infectious adults and preventing its spread throughout the household and the community are important strategies for reducing children's exposure to TB.

Like adults, children with HIV are more vulnerable to TB. For example, in 1990 in Lusaka, Zambia, 37 percent of the children who were admitted to the hospital with TB were also HIV-positive. By 1991, this number had increased to 56 percent, and by 1992, it had jumped to 68.9 percent (World Health Organization, 2001). Diagnosis of TB, already a difficult process in children, is even harder when HIV is also present. As a result, some children are falsely diagnosed as TB-positive and given treatment they do not need, while others who actually have TB may be missed and not receive any treatment at all. The high prevalence of HIV in many developing countries, in all age groups, leaves children in these populations especially susceptible to the vagaries of TB.

In households where family members have TB, children are vulnerable to direct exposure as well as to indirect influences from the disease. Beyond the potential of becoming infected, children in poor households that have TB are at increased risk of additional burdens due to the loss of parental income or the accumulation of debt. A cycle of lifelong impairment may begin when loss of family income leads to malnourishment in children, which increases susceptibility to TB as well as overall health and education disadvantages. Children who suffer from poor nutrition and ill health have below average school enrollment and attendance, and lower educational achievement. Lack of education is correlated with inferior access to health care services, which is in turn related to an increased risk of developing TB. Circumstances in childhood begin a cycle of TB risk and consequences that may persist across the life span.

In families where the primary caregiver is ill or preoccupied with caring for other family members who are ill, even healthy children may be affected by TB through inadvertent neglect or disregard. Children in developing countries become especially vulnerable if their mother, more so than their father, becomes sick and dies. Statistics show that survival of the mother is strongly correlated with the survival of a child up to the age of 10 years. For example, in Bangladesh, the death rate of children is increased by 6 children per 100,000 for both boys and girls when a father dies. When a mother dies, however, the death rate of children is increased by 50 sons per 100,000 children and 144 daughters per 100,000 children (World Health Organization, 2001). In the best of circumstances, children are among the most vulnerable members of society; when TB is a factor in the life of children, they are susceptible to the direct threat of the disease, as well as to the indirect social consequences that accompany it.

Migration and Immigration

Migration, the regular movement of a group of people from one location to another, is a social phenomenon that is related to several factors, including poverty, the need to obtain seasonal work, and the search for food. Two-thirds of migration flows occur in developing countries. Conflict and war, natural disasters, and political upheaval also cause people to flee to new locations because of fear of political or ethnic persecution. Migrants and refugees may share an increased TB risk because of lack of access to decent housing, overcrowded conditions, lack of food, and inadequate health care. Beyond the initially increased risks of TB associated with relocation, when migrants or refugees eventually reach their next destination, regardless of how affluent a new location may be in general, impoverished circumstances are likely to relegate them to the same social and economic conditions they left behind. Poverty, overcrowding, substandard housing, poor sanitation, and lack of access to medical services tend to follow migratory groups. Language difficulties, unfamiliarity with the customs and culture of a new place, racism, and fear of immigration authorities can be additional barriers for people trying to establish themselves in new countries.

Since people often emigrate from areas with high levels of social deprivation and high endemic TB, immigrant populations have a high risk of bringing the disease with them to a new location. Additionally, the impoverished circumstances that often await them in a new country increase the risk of acquiring new TB infection because of continuing socioeconomic disadvantage and proximity to other people who are already infected. For example, in 2000, almost one-fourth of the people with TB in east London had arrived in the United Kingdom within the previous year (World Health Organization, 2001).

In the United States, a common form of migration involves the seasonal influx of migrant workers. The transient nature of migrant work, coupled with the long duration of TB treatment, makes it difficult for seasonal workers to balance their need to work with the need to take care of their health. Some states have set up effective voluntary TB screening programs for migrant farm workers. The state of Virginia, for example, has made a significant effort to obtain reliable follow-up information (such as travel itineraries, winter addresses, and addresses of relatives) for workers who have started TB treatment for latent or active infection following screening. Of migrant farm workers who were tested on the east and west coasts of the United States, between 31 and 47 percent tested positive for TB, and were considered six times more likely than the general population of employed workers to develop TB (World Health Organization, 2001). The high incidence of TB among immigrants and migrant workers has led many developed countries to enact more active screening programs in these populations. Additionally, efforts are being made to provide better TB treatment and follow-up care in migrant and immigrant populations since these people are frequently among the most disenfranchised members of society.

3

The History of Tuberculosis

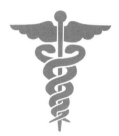

TB has existed since ancient times. Its history consists of a complicated pattern of repetitive appearances and disappearances throughout time, but a lack of definite facts and documentation makes it difficult to put all the pieces together. Known by various names in different historical eras, TB has always been a disease that was influenced by the social, medical, and intellectual sensibilities of the time and, in turn, its presence influenced the human race. The history of TB may perhaps be best illustrated through narrative accounts of some of the people and societies that suffered with it and eventually learned to cure it. Across the centuries, TB has left its mark on the world.

TUBERCULOSIS IN ANCIENT CIVILIZATIONS

In spite of some uncertainty about how common TB has been throughout history, evidence that TB existed in ancient times has been well documented. Burial grounds from the last part of the Stone Age have produced skeletal remains bearing evidence that TB affected prehistoric man 6,000 years ago. Excavations of mummified bodies from the tombs of ancient Egypt have unearthed both microscopic and visible evidence of widespread TB disease from that era. Physical deformities characteristic of TB in the spine were depicted in the drawings, pottery, and statues of ancient Egypt as early as 3000 B.C.E. (Before the Common Era). As humans began to migrate and populate the world, evidence from archeology, ancient language, art, and literature suggests that TB made the journey to geographical areas as far reaching as the Americas, the Nile Valley, China, India, and Western Europe.

In ancient and biblical writings, phthisis and consumption are commonly referenced, and descriptions of a pulmonary disease that seemed to devour the afflicted person from within are frequent. Even in the most ancient legal texts, formulated by Hammurabi in 1948 and 1905 B.C.E. and engraved on a stone pillar, there is mention of a chronic lung disease, which in all probability refers to TB. Modern autopsy investigations of ancient remains have found the telltale pulmonary cavities and lesions left by TB, indicating that it was an important disease in ancient civilizations. Even bacteriological evidence of TB in ancient times exists in the form of acid-fast bacteria found in smears taken from a lesion on a very well-preserved mummy of a child from around 700 B.C.E. While physical evidence documents the existence of TB in antiquity, its importance must have varied from civilization to civilization if its frequency can be inferred from the

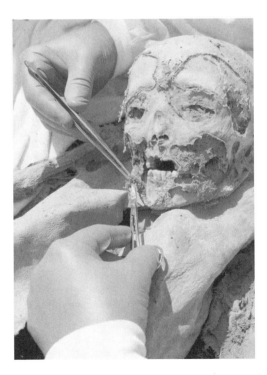

Hungarian professor of microbiology Karoly Nagy takes tissue samples from a mummy in the Hungarian Natural History Museum in Budapest, Hungary, in 2007. The museum stores 265 mummies and offered tissue samples from each of them for Nagy's research. Scientists found that most of the deceased had been infected by TB. AP Photo/Bela Szandelszky.

writings of ancient scholars. Without explanation or justification, and lacking effective treatments to control it, TB mushroomed and receded across ancient times and places in a characteristic pattern of occurrence that would persist for centuries.

In ancient Greece and Rome, physicians began to separate the field of medicine from the worlds of religion and superstition, and they wrote about the disease now known as TB. As a more knowledge-based approach to disease developed, these doctors were responsible for bringing valuable insight to the historical presence of TB. The concept of phthisis, an early name for TB, appears in Greek literature around this time. Much has been learned about the occurrence of TB in ancient Greece from the writings of Hippocrates (460–375 B.C.E.), the physician who is called the father of medicine. He believed that TB was caused by growths in the lungs, which he called *tubercula*. Recognizing that TB was often a fatal disease, he wrote at length about various forms of the disease and described characteristic symptoms and signs that are still associated with TB today—fevers, sweats, cough, and wasting away. Hippocrates warned his fellow physicians to stay away from patients with advanced phthisis since they would invariably die and ruin the reputation of the physician who was caring for them. Knowing nothing about the existence of microorganisms or the mechanisms of infectious disease, Hippocrates considered pulmonary phthisis to be a hereditary condition and other healers followed his lead.

Alexandria, a city near the Nile River on the coast of Egypt, was an ancient center for scholarly pursuits and the place where the greatest Greek physicians of the day practiced the art of medicine. Aretæus was a Cappadocian monk and a Greek physician who lived in Alexandria at the beginning of the second century C.E. (in the Common Era). He added to the body of knowledge regarding ancient TB through his writings and vivid descriptions, and he influenced the perception of the disease going forward in history. Aretæus was the first to suggest that a specific body type was associated with TB, noting that a person who was prone to the disease was more likely to be pale and to have a slender, weak body. His mistaken belief that a certain body type was associated with the likelihood of developing TB persisted for many centuries. He described pulmonary consumption (another early name for TB) as a disease with a generally poor prognosis that was characterized by chronic discharge of opaque, whitish-yellow fluid from the lungs.

Even a century later, as Roman influence spread over Europe and the Middle East, Greek physicians continued to be at the forefront of medicine. Galen (131–202 C.E.), a Greek physician who went to Rome in 162 C.E., continued to record the history of TB. Even though he had no knowledge of the concepts of infection or contagion, he veered away from the idea that consumption was related to hereditary considerations, believing instead that TB could be spread from person to

---

A Description of Advanced Tuberculosis by Aretæus

"Voice hoarse, neck slightly bent, tender and stiff; fingers slender but joints swollen; severe wasting of the fleshy parts leaving the bones prominently outlined;...The nose is sharp and slender, the cheeks are prominent and abnormally flushed; the eyes are deeply sunk in the hollows but brilliant and glittering;...The slender parts of the jaws rests on the teeth as if smiling but it is the smile of cadavers....The muscles of the limbs all wasted....The shoulder blades are the wings of the birds."

From the *Causes and Symptoms of Chronic Diseases* (translation published in 1856 by the Sydenham Society, London, UK).

---

person. He recognized TB in its many forms and warned against intimate contact with people known to have the disease. Galen was one of the first to conjecture that TB might have an infectious quality, a concept that would prove to be both prophetic and correct. For treatment, he recommended simple remedies like fresh air, high altitudes, and dry climates.

TUBERCULOSIS IN EUROPE: THE MIDDLE AGES THROUGH THE 18TH CENTURY

Throughout the Middle Ages, the period of time between the collapse of the Roman Empire and the beginning of the European Renaissance around the year 1300, TB was apparently not a common illness, although it did exist in some forms. The Renaissance, a French word that literally means rebirth, was a cultural movement that began in Florence, Italy, in the Late Middle Ages and later spread to the rest of Europe. During this time of artistic and intellectual expansion, new ideas about disease and medicine were also formulated. Picking up where the ancient ideas of Galen left off, Girolamo Frascatoro (1478–1553), an Italian physician, poet, and astronomer, advanced his theory that diseases were caused by "seed-like elements" that could transmit infection over distance. Far ahead of his time and well before the acceptance of a germ theory of disease, Frascatoro hypothesized in his work called *De contagione* that phthisis was transmitted by invisible particles called *seminaria* and that it could survive on the clothes of a consumptive patient for two years. He also developed the premise that phthisis came from a lung ulcer, an idea that is considered to be a major step forward in the description of consumption and its nature as an infectious condition. Frascatoro noted that, beginning in the Greek tradition of medicine, the word "phthisis" had been used as a catch-all expression to describe all manners of wasting illness. To clarify the subject, Frascatoro advocated reserving phthisis to describe only pulmonary consumption.

The anatomy and pathology of disease in general began to be more closely investigated in the 16th century. With the development of the printing press by Johannes Gutenburg, newly obtained medical knowledge circulated more rapidly among the great minds of the time than it had before. A greater understanding of the normal physiology of the human body was advanced by Andreas Vesalius (1514–1564), the eminent Renaissance anatomist, physician, and author. He and other physicians began developing techniques to perform postmortem examinations (also known as autopsies) so they could study the human body after death. Physicians began to make a connection between the condition of the body during autopsy and the cause of death, and an understanding of the symptoms of specific diseases and their effect on the body began to be formulated. This was the age during which a detailed anatomical and pathological description of consumption began to emerge.

Fransiscus de la Boë, better known as Sylvius (1614–1672), was a professor of clinical and anatomical medicine in Holland. His expertise attracted students from every part of Europe, and it was Sylvius who decisively associated the characteristic nodules in the lungs and other organs with phthisis. He called them *tubercles* and described their progression to cavities and ulcers. Two of Sylvius's students also added to the early body of knowledge about phthisis. Thomas Willis (1621–1675) related the localized lesions in the lungs of tuberculous patients to the general wasting away of the body as a whole. In addition, he described various types of the disease, including chronic TB, with characteristic periods of worsening and remission, and miliary or "galloping" TB. Galloping TB earned its name because of the sudden onset and very rapid course of illness, which caused extensive destruction of lung tissue in just a few short months. Richard Morton (1637–1698), another of Sylvius's students, described three stages of phthisis: initial inflammation, the formation of tubercles, and the ultimate progression to ulcers and full-blown consumption. Both Sylvius and Morton also identified a syndrome, which they believed was a combination of phthisis and a skin disease, called scrofula.

In realty, scrofula is a form of TB that affects the lymph glands of the neck, causing them to become painlessly swollen and rubbery. Much can be inferred about TB during the 1600s from the frequent descriptions of rituals that were held for the healing of scrofula. This condition was such a common presentation of TB during this period that the healing of scrofula became the focus of a ceremony in the royal courts of Europe. In these societies, where kings and queens were believed to have a divine authority granted to them by God, touching ceremonies were conducted to heal a variety of diseases, most notably scrofula. Many

Shakespeare's Description of the Healing Power of the Royal Touch:
***Macbeth* (Act IV, scene 3)**

"What's the disease he means?"...
"Tis call'd the evil....How he solicits heaven,
Himself best knows: but strangely-visited people,
All swoln and ulcerous, pitiful to the eye,
The mere despair of surgery, he cures,
Hanging a golden stamp about their necks,
Put on with holy prayers: and 'tis spoken,
To the succeeding royalty he leaves
The healing benediction."

generations of European monarchs "cured" scrofula by praying and touching crowds of patients, many who had traveled for miles to receive the royal caress and a traditional gold coin. The ritual to cure scrofula, also known as the King's Evil, provides historical context for presence of TB in medieval Europe.

Next to William Shakespeare, Samuel Johnson (1709–1784) is perhaps the most quoted writer of English. His influence and contributions to the English language through his work as a poet, essayist, and novelist are so substantial that the later part of the 18th century in English-speaking countries is sometimes simply called the Age of Johnson. After nine years of continuous work, he completed *A Dictionary of the English Language*, a book that had a great impact and has been described as one of the greatest scholarly achievements of all time. Published in 1755, the *Dictionary* brought Johnson popularity and success, and until the completion of the *Oxford English Dictionary* 150 years later, Johnson's work was considered the most important British book of its kind.

At a very young age, Johnson contracted scrofula. It inflamed his lymph glands and spread to his optic and auditory nerves, leaving him deaf in the left ear and almost blind in one eye. When he was two and a half years old, his mother took him on a long journey from his home in rural England to London, where he and 200 other scrofulous patients participated in a touching ceremony performed by Queen Anne. Did the royal touch heal scrofula? Apparently not in Johnson's case—several years later he underwent surgery to drain the infected lymph nodes, and although he was disfigured by the procedure, the scrofula subsequently healed and Johnson was not further affected by TB.

Belief in the power of the royal touch may perhaps best be explained by the nature of scrofula—it is a condition that usually causes little pain and ultimately resolves spontaneously, with no need for actual medical treatment. Additionally,

> Hope is necessary in every condition.
>
> —Samuel Johnson

once a person recovers from scrofula, some immunity to other forms of TB may even develop. Without other evidence to support a high incidence of TB at this time, the common occurrence of scrofula in late medieval Europe can only suggest that TB in other forms was also prevalent. Not surprisingly, the divine authority of kings and queens did not enable them to cure TB and, in fact, it did not protect them from contracting it either. In 1643, at 42 years of age, King Louis XIII of France died of consumption.

In spite of the fact that the prevailing opinion of the day asserted that TB was a hereditary condition, medical literature from the 17th century provides clear-cut evidence that some physicians and politicians were convinced that it was a contagious disease. In 1699, the Italian Republic of Lucca issued a proclamation that "human health must no longer be endangered by objects remaining after the death of a consumptive person" and the possessions of people who had died of TB were ordered to be burned. Physicians were urged to perform postmortem examinations on patients who were believed to have had phthisis and the names of patients with consumption were supposed to be reported to authorities. Fear of contagion became contagious. In Vienna, Austria, a physician reported seeing a man fall over dead from having stepped in sputum expectorated by a man with consumption. Another patient was reported to have contracted TB from breathing in fumes released from smoldering sputum that had been discarded on burning coal. A published description of TB being transmitted through the dying kiss between a consumptive wife and her grieving husband offers further evidence that the theory of contagion had some early support. In Prague, in the modern day Czech Republic, there were strict quarantine regulations for patients with consumption. Despite these indications that the concept of TB contagion had begun to nip at the heels of traditional medical wisdom, the prevailing belief during the 17th century and for many years thereafter maintained that TB was caused by a weak hereditary constitution, aggravated by an unwholesome lifestyle.

At the beginning of the 18th century, further insight into the nature of TB was gained through the inventive work of Benjamin Marten. An English physician with great curiosity, Marten began to wonder if TB really could be passed from one person to another. To explore the notion, he used the earlier work of Antonie van Leeuwenhoek, the pioneering microbiologist who discovered the microscope, as his guide. During his experiments into the nature of TB, Marten became the first person to observe and describe single-celled microorganisms. In 1720, he published a groundbreaking work called *A New Theory of Consumptions, More especially of a Phthisis or Consumption of the Lungs,* in which he speculated that pulmonary TB might be caused by "wonderfully minute living creatures" or a "certain species of *Animalculae,*" the word he coined to describe the tiny life forms he saw under his makeshift lens.

Marten wondered if the small creatures he observed could enter the body and produce the lesions and symptoms of phthisis. He stated that, while phthisis might indeed be the product of inheritance, it might also be possible that it was transmitted by person-to-person contact. Although he didn't believe that occasional association with a consumptive person was necessarily harmful, he cautioned that continuous contact was dangerous, especially for persons with limited resistance, such as parents of children with phthisis. He observed that frequently eating with a consumptive person or conversing in close enough proximity that exhaled consumptive air could enter the lungs of a healthy person might be ways in which the disease spread. These very specific insights into the infectious nature of TB were both astonishing and extraordinarily accurate for someone who only possessed the limited knowledge of his day. Although Marten's book would not become well regarded for another 150 years, his suspicion that tiny creatures might be responsible for TB foreshadowed the discoveries that ushered in the germ theory of infectious disease.

TUBERCULOSIS IN 19TH-CENTURY EUROPE

In 19th-century Europe, the numbers tell the tale of another precipitous rise in the incidence of TB: in the early part of the century, 36 percent of all recorded deaths at one Paris hospital were due to TB; in London, approximately 6 percent of all deaths reported between 1831 and 1835 were caused by TB; a physician estimated that one fourth of the English population had TB in 1815; and in the 1830s, 30 percent of deaths among English laborers were due to TB (Daniel, 1997). During the years of the Industrial Revolution in Europe, TB relentlessly savaged the emerging working class. The heavy burdens of industrialization— poverty, malnutrition, and overcrowded, putrid living conditions—created the perfect environment for TB to kill en masse. Industrialization occurred at different times in different places in Europe, but TB was its steady companion because the changing economic system created compromised social conditions for the workers. In England, an explosive increase in the number of cases of TB occurred between 1790 and 1850. In places such as France, Germany, Scandinavia, and Eastern Europe, an onslaught of TB occurred later or for longer periods of time depending on the nature of industrialization in each location.

Workers such as seamstresses, bakers, printers, and shoemakers who often labored in crowded and poorly ventilated sweatshops were the perfect targets of consumption. Child labor became commonplace in the factories of England around 1800. Long hours of work in closed, crowded, filthy factories, poor nutrition, and shared beds for sleeping most certainly gave tubercle bacilli no end of attractive hosts to prey upon. TB thrived where poverty, inhumane working conditions, inhumane living conditions, and grime flourished. However, the damage inflicted by TB in 19th-century Europe was not reserved for the working class of an industrializing continent; TB ravaged the scholarly as well as the unskilled and claimed many victims from the young, aristocratic intellectuals of this generation. The artistic potential of a generation was devastated as many literary and artistic careers came to untimely ends at the hands of TB.

While detailed stories from the ranks of the poor may have been largely overlooked by history, the fates of the literary greats of the Romantic Age have been well documented. The Brontës were a prominent literary family whose suffering at the hands of TB is a typical story of the time rather than a portrayal of a singular artistic tragedy. Charlotte, Emily, and Anne were gifted authors who wrote several novels that are considered great works of English literature. However, as was the case with so many artists of the day, intelligence and talent proved to be no match for TB. After the death of their mother, it was too difficult for their clergyman father and an aunt to care for the six Brontë children so the four oldest sisters, Maria, Elizabeth, Charlotte, and Emily, were sent to live at a boarding school. During their time at school, the girls were likely exposed to TB and within a year it began to take its ugly toll on the family. In 1825, 12-year-old Maria and 11-year-old Elizabeth became the first two siblings to die of TB. Between 1847 and 1849, following the publication of Charlotte's book *Jane Eyre*, Emily's book *Wuthering Heights*, and Anne's book *Agnes Grey*, Emily, Anne, and their brother Branwell became the next three Brontë siblings to die from TB. Charlotte, the last living sibling, published two more books and in June 1854, she married and became pregnant. Soon after, her health took a dramatic turn for the worse and on March 31, 1855, at the young age of 38, Charlotte and her unborn child died. Her death certificate lists the cause of death as phthisis. In the course of 30 years, six Brontë siblings died of TB; this tragic family story is historically significant both in light of the literary talent that was devastated and by virtue of the disease that killed them all.

As TB consumed all classes of European society during the Romantic Age, the pale, thin, fragile look of TB became perversely immortalized as the idealized standard of beauty. Perhaps less able to cope with the harsh reality of desolation and disease than their working-class counterparts, the artists and writers of 19th-century Europe transformed the ugly reality of TB into a romanticized destiny. Helpless to prevent the havoc inflicted by TB, numerous consumptive poets and writers instead embraced the suffering and ultimately began to regard it as a breeding ground for creative genius. The sickly look of TB was artistically portrayed in statues and paintings, and was characterized in works of literature. In pace with the medical knowledge of the day, the suffering, young talents believed that TB was particularly attracted to the sensitive temperaments of those who practiced the Romantic arts. As a result, the image of tuberculous beauty was even sought after by healthy members of 19th-century upper-class society. TB, art, illness, sentimentality, beauty, creativity, and death became inextricably intertwined during the Romantic Age.

Ultimately known as the most fragile and sensitive of the Romantic poets, John Keats (1795–1821) became more famous for his early death from TB than for his dynamic life. A trained physician, Keats began to write poetry during his hospital training. His poems were well received by literary circles in London, and by the end of his medical training Keats had decided that poetry, not medicine, was his calling. After caring for his consumptive brother, Keats experienced the first sign that his vigorous good health was about to be challenged by TB when he coughed up blood. Under the care of doctors, Keats was treated in the typical manner of the day—he underwent bloodletting to remove the evil tempers from his body, his doctors confined him to bed in a closed and airless room, he was put on a starvation diet, he took sea voyages so that he could be exposed to the restorative powers of the fresh air, and he was encouraged to take gentle horseback rides.

Growing increasingly weak and ever more ill, he continued to write poems. In spite of the general belief that TB produced more creativity, sensitivity, and sentimentality, after he became ill Keats never again produced the exceptional quality of work he had exhibited in his earlier poems. Once TB claimed him, Keats's decline was swift and unremitted; he never regained his health and the Romantic conviction that a creative mind could triumph over a diseased body was seriously challenged. For Keats, TB was a particularly overwhelming and severe disease; it would take only 11 months from the first recognition of TB symptoms for him to die of the disease. An autopsy examination revealed that his lungs were almost entirely destroyed, indicating that the disease process had probably started long before Keats knew that he had TB. Keats and his frail, consumptive, wispy silhouette became the epitome of the Romantic obsession that ironically made TB a disease associated with sentimentality and beauty.

Nineteenth-century sentiment eventually gave way to a realism that recognized the misery and suffering of TB. As Romantic ideas about TB expired, the disease began to be regarded more accurately as a blight of industrialization, a

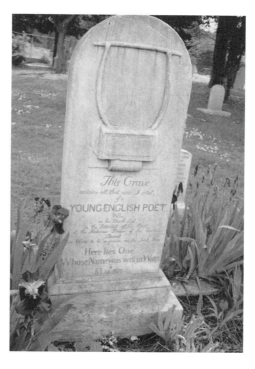

The tombstone of John Keats in the Protestant Cemetery, Rome. The inscription reads: "This grave contains all that was Mortal, of a YOUNG ENGLISH POET, Who on his Death Bed, in the Bitterness of his Heart, at the Malicious Power of his Enemies, Desired these Words to be engraved on his Tomb Stone 'Here lies One Whose Name was writ in Water' Feb 24th 1821." Picture by Giovanni Dall'Orto, March 31, 2008.

"Here lies One Whose Name was writ in Water"

John Keats was the personification of the Romantic identity that was attached to TB during the 19th century. Keats died on February 24, 1821, less than one year after noticing blood on his pillow, the first symptom that he had TB. On his deathbed, he uttered these last words: "I shall die easy... Thank God it has come" before dying peacefully in his sleep. He had told a friend that he did not want his name to appear on his tombstone—that he wished only to be commemorated with the line "Here lies One Whose Name was writ in Water." These words appeared in Keats's *Poetic Works* (1821), and they refer to the fleeting nature of fame and life itself. The rest of the tombstone inscription was added by close friends who nursed him through his illness, and were grief-stricken and bitter about the harsh way that Keats's poetry had been treated by the critics.

symbol of social inequities, and a consequence of economic hardships. Once TB was no longer identified as the inspiration of the literary elite and aristocrats, it began to be truthfully regarded as the mass killer and source of human suffering that it was during the 19th century in Europe.

THE HISTORY OF TUBERCULOSIS IN THE UNITED STATES

Although its presence in early America is documented, TB was apparently not a scourge of epic proportions there as it was in Egypt and Europe. Remains from burial grounds have yielded evidence that TB existed among the early people of the Ohio and Mississippi River valleys, but TB does not appear to have been common among Native Americans in the West or in the Arctic until after contact with European colonists.

When the American colonies were settled, there is little doubt, but also little direct evidence, that TB made the voyage from England with the Pilgrims. Half of the Pilgrims who reached Plymouth, Massachusetts, in 1620 died during their first winter in the New World. Although some authors have suggested that TB may have swept through the colony, there were no physicians among the colonists and no definitive evidence exists to support the TB theory. Alternately, others theorize that the brisk climate and fresh air of New England were protective against the spread of TB since the disease appears to have been much less common in New England than it was in England during this period.

It may never be known for certain whether TB was responsible for widespread death in Plymouth or if the climate protected the settlers from it, but it is a fact that the colonies did not totally escape TB. Cotton Mather (1663–1728), a prominent New England Puritan who became well known for his role in the Salem Witch Trials, probably had TB. He and several other writers of the period described several clear-cut cases of TB. By the time of the Revolutionary War, TB was a well-established disease in the colonies and accounted for approximately one out of every five to seven deaths in New England (Daniel, 1997).

By the early 1800s, most Americans had firsthand familiarity with TB, the deadliest disease in America in the first half of the 19th century. As in Europe, both popular opinion and the medical expertise of the day supported the notion that TB was hereditary. The family members of people who had TB were believed to have a predisposition toward developing the disease themselves. Since multiple cases of TB frequently occurred in one family, the theory that inherited health traits influenced the likelihood of developing the disease seemed probable. It was generally believed that little could be done for those born with a predisposition toward TB, so supportive care and a balmy climate were all that

---

TB in New England

By the beginning of the 19th century, TB was a well-known and feared disease in America. During this time, TB was recorded as the cause of 23 percent of the deaths in Salem, Massachusetts, 27 percent of the deaths in Brookline, Massachusetts, and 20 percent to 25 percent of the deaths in New York City (Daniel, 1997).

---

was generally recommended to those who showed signs of consumptive illness. Henry David Thoreau (1817–1862), the American author and naturalist best known for his book *Walden; or, Life in the Woods*, was a member of a consumptive family. When he died at the age of 45, he was only one of several family members to succumb to TB.

The family of Ralph Waldo Emerson (1803–1882) is a portrait of TB across the generations. Emerson was a well-known essayist, philosopher, and poet whose teachings and oration greatly influenced American thought in the mid-1880s. The Emerson family immigrated to the New World from England in 1638. During their first 100 years in Massachusetts, there is no evidence of the occurrence of TB in the family. Then, in 1811, when consumption was the most frequently recognized cause of death in New England, Reverend William Emerson died of TB at the age of 42. Ralph Waldo, one of his surviving sons, developed TB but overcame the acute form of the disease and lived to the age of 79. However, TB would continue to leave its mark on many other members of the family for generations to come, starting with three of Emerson's brothers. His oldest brother showed signs of pulmonary disease in early adulthood and suffered from episodes of illness throughout his life, and two other brothers died of galloping consumption, a very aggressive form of the disease. In 1829, Emerson married a woman with active TB. Shortly after their marriage, her health began a precipitous decline that led to her death in 1831. While the death of Emerson's wife marked an unfortunate end for her, it was not the end of TB in the Emerson family. Modern research into the genealogy of the Emersons has documented subsequent deaths from TB and clinical cases of the disease through at least 10 more generations of the family. The frequency of multiple cases of TB in one family, like the Emersons, bolstered the theory that bad inherited health traits biased the likelihood that a person would develop the disease.

From the 1840s through the 1880s, TB played a role in westward migration, as people with symptoms of the disease sought respite in places they believed to be conducive to better health. Then, even though no real cure was at hand, the occurrence of TB in America began to decline. While the incidence of TB in

Europe is thought to have peaked around 1850, in America the worst of 19th-century TB was probably over a little sooner. Theories about why TB began to decline in the America are inconclusive, but better nutrition, the practice of confining sick people, and the development of widespread immunity after extensive exposure within communities may have all played a role. Although the early history of TB was probably more dramatic in Europe than in America, the disease undoubtedly left a mark on the American psyche and influenced the concept of infectious disease. At the beginning of the 20th century, surveys suggest that almost all adults in European and American cities were TB positive, indicating that almost everyone had been infected with TB at some point in time.

4

Early Efforts to Tame Tuberculosis

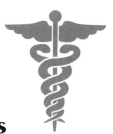

The march of TB through time is also a story of medical and scientific progression toward a cure. Centuries would pass during which doctors could recognize the symptoms of TB but could do little to stop its spread or offer a cure. In 1882, when German microbiologist Robert Koch proved that *M. tuberculosis* was the indisputable cause of TB, a significant milestone was reached. However, it would be another 50 years before the cure for TB would be discovered, leaving a huge void during which uncertainty, isolation, and guesswork formed the basis of treatment. The discovery of an antibiotic that could kill TB bacteria without being too toxic to the patient forever changed the treatment of TB. Until that time, however, observing patients and studying every detail of their symptoms helped physicians gain a greater understanding of the disease process, led to new techniques of examination, and began to unravel some of the mysteries of TB.

HEARING THE SOUNDS OF TUBERCULOSIS

To effectively treat a disease, accurate assessment of a patient's physical condition is necessary. Without the necessary tools or clinical knowledge to inform their judgment, early physicians were limited to their powers of observation and the influence of popular opinion to guide TB treatment. Since TB is most frequently a disease of the lungs, doctors treating sick patients began to notice that different sounds heard in the chest were related to different characteristics of the disease. This was the beginning of a diagnostic revolution that would transform how TB was treated.

Early in the evolution of TB treatment, an astute physician named Leopold Auenbrugger (1722–1809) noticed that tapping the chest of a patient produced a variety of sounds that depended on the condition of the patient's lungs. Using his musically trained ear, he began to associate the different sounds he heard with different symptoms he observed in his patient. By interpreting the sounds, Auenbrugger began to gain valuable information about the specific condition of a patient's lungs. These observations became the foundation of the examination technique known as percussion, a practice still used by physicians today.

Auenbrugger began to recognize and understand different resonance of sounds in the chest. To evaluate a patient's condition, he determined if the same sounds came from both lungs and noticed how a sound changed in relation to the position of the patient's body. To refine the accuracy of his interpretation of the chest sounds, Auenbrugger compared patient lung condition during autopsy evaluation with the findings he had obtained during percussion. Even though percussion is a simple procedure that was first practiced as early as the late 1700s, for a long time the slowly evolving medical establishment did not understand its value or routinely use it to assess the condition of TB patients. Eventually, the sounds of percussion were added to the powers of observation, and physicians began to treat patients on the basis of information from inside as well outside the patient's body.

Knowledge of how the sounds of TB were related to the stage of the disease was greatly advanced by a doctor named René Théophile Hyacinthe Laënnec (1781–1826). His great contribution to TB was the revolutionary idea that different stages of pulmonary TB were different presentations of a single disease process and that the different forms of TB were really different aspects of pulmonary TB, not entirely different diseases. Laënnec was also responsible for inventing one of the most valuable and commonly used medical tools in history, the stethoscope. In 1816, while examining a rather chubby patient, Laënnec realized that percussion and directly listening to the chest were useless because the patient's layer of fat muffled the sounds. Using a principle of acoustics that he remembered from games he had played as a child, Laënnec rolled up a piece of paper to make a hollow tube and put one end on his patient's chest and the other to his ear. Through the tube, Laënnec could hear the distinct and clear sounds of a beating heart and breathing.

Early models of the stethoscope were one-ear versions instead of the two-ear type that is used today. With the help of his makeshift listening devices, Laënnec

---

The Bacteria Lives Longer Than the Patient

In these early years, it wasn't known that TB was caused by a microorganism or that the bacteria could survive in dead tissue for weeks or months, and retain the capacity to infect again. Without this knowledge, Laënnec took few safety precautions when he performed autopsy examinations on patients who had died from TB. As a result, he became infected with TB while handling and examining highly infectious tissue specimens. Ironically, Laënnec was diagnosed with the help of the stethoscope that he discovered and he died of TB, the disease that he had helped to fingerprint. Before he died, he bequeathed his stethoscope to his nephew, saying that this innovation was his greatest legacy.

---

was able to describe a variety of lung diseases, including TB, by the sounds they produced. As was usually the case with innovative ideas, the new technique of indirect listening was initially greeted with skepticism by the medical establishment. Within a few years, however, the value of being able to clearly hear what was going on inside the human body was recognized, and stethoscopes, mostly of the homemade variety, began to be accepted as an indispensible tool of the trade. Their use greatly advanced the process of diagnosing TB and other lung diseases.

SEEING INSIDE THE HUMAN BODY—
THE DISCOVERY OF X-RAYS

The diagnosis and assessment of TB was greatly advanced by the invention of the stethoscope and the ability to hear what was going on inside the body. Did anyone dare to dream about being able to see what was going on inside the body? Like many other important scientific breakthroughs, x-ray was discovered purely by accident. In 1895, Wilhelm Konrad von Röntgen (1845–1923), a physics professor at a Bavarian university, was in the process of completing an experiment using electricity. As he was investigating what happened when an electric current was passed through a vacuum tube surrounded by black cardboard, he noticed a mysterious fluorescent glow in the darkened laboratory. Out of curiosity, he investigated the strange effect and discovered that it was caused by rays that were able to penetrate the cardboard shield. To his surprise, all the objects he placed in the path of the newly discovered rays became transparent. Eventually, he raised his hand into the path of the rays and became the first person to see human bones visibly outlined beneath the skin. He christened the newly discovered rays "x-rays." Unlike so many other advances that initially received lukewarm receptions in the medical world, x-rays were immediately proclaimed as revolutionary and scientists went to work to improve the fledgling technology.

Within months of the discovery of x-rays, the first fluoroscopes were created and physicians were able to obtain real-time moving images of the internal structures of a patient. In its simplest form, a fluoroscope consists of an x-ray source and a fluorescent screen; the patient is placed between these two pieces of equipment. Early fluoroscopes were simply cardboard funnels that were open at the narrow end so the observer could look. The wide end was closed with a thin cardboard piece that had been coated on the inside with a layer of fluorescent metal salt. Images obtained with these crude techniques were faint and difficult to interpret, but the great inventor Thomas Edison quickly discovered that calcium tungstate screens produced brighter images. He is credited with designing and producing the first commercially available fluoroscope. By the 1920s, the usefulness of chest x-rays and fluoroscopy to help diagnose and assess TB was well established. With the availability of x-ray images, doctors were finally able to gauge the severity of TB when it was initially diagnosed and to monitor its subsequent progression.

THE TUBERCULIN SKIN TEST—HUMAN AND BOVINE TUBERCULOSIS

After Koch discovered the cause of TB and announced it to the world in 1882, he retreated from the public spotlight and had little more to say about TB until 1900. At this time, Koch reappeared to declare that he had identified a substance that could protect against or, in some cases, even cure TB. The material he had discovered was tuberculin, a substance that he extracted from tubercle bacilli. Although it did not live up to the original hype—tuberculin could neither cure TB nor protect against it—Koch recognized its potential value when he realized that tuberculin actually caused a negative reaction in some patients. A response to tuberculin was indicative that an immune response was occurring, which meant that M. *tuberculosis* was lurking, even if no symptoms were identifiable. The ability to identify the presence of TB before symptoms were apparent held great diagnostic potential. A reaction to tuberculin was used as the basis for developing a TB skin test.

Veterinarians were the first to use tuberculin as a tool to diagnose TB in animals. Bovine TB was a huge problem in cattle, and the danger of transmission from cows to humans through the drinking of unpasteurized milk was a widely recognized threat to public health. Although *Mycobacterium bovis* almost never causes pulmonary TB, it appears to have been the cause of approximately 15 percent of deaths from TB in Europe around 1900. TB caused by the bovine strain of bacteria usually presents as intestinal TB, a painful and potentially fatal condition in children. Intestinal TB frequently requires surgeries to relieve intestinal obstructions, and it can progress to malnutrition and general weakness that are severe enough to cause death. Bovine TB was entirely preventable for 50 years before the development of antibiotic treatment for TB, and it now only occurs in places where the problem has not been actively addressed.

When skin testing shows that a cow has TB, it is removed from the herd and destroyed to protect other animals and humans from infection. Within a decade of initiating skin tests to identify TB in cows in the United States, 300 million tests were performed, approximately 4 million of them were positive, and cash payments were made to the cattle owners to reimburse them for their losses (Dormandy, 2001). In 1937 alone, payments totaling $27 million were paid to cattle owners, but the necessity and effectiveness of these measures were never questioned in the United States. Between 1910 and 1932, the death rate from milk-borne TB decreased by two-thirds in New York and by 91 percent in Massachusetts. By 1940, all states except California reported that 99 percent of their milk cows were TB-free, and California only missed the 99 percent mark by a small margin. This remarkable progress in the pursuit of public health in the United States was not matched by advances in Europe, where bovine TB remained rampant in many countries.

Some countries in Europe acted quickly to control the threat of bovine TB. Denmark, Finland, Germany, Italy, Switzerland, Belgium, France, Holland, Norway, and Sweden all had rules in place to govern bovine TB control by 1914. Even though the need to clean up the milk supply in Britain had been long recognized, there was intense resistance to initiating preventive measures to control bovine TB and make the milk supply safe. In 1847, the medical journal *The Lancet* reported that it was difficult to find milk in London that was not contaminated by microscopic blood or pus.

In England, most veterinarians who worked in academics supported measures for enforced inspection of cows, removal of sick cows from the herd, milk pasteurization, and any other steps deemed necessary to stop bovine TB. However, veterinarians who worked in the field had a different motivation where bovine TB was concerned. Practicing veterinarians resisted all bovine TB control measures because they depended on the goodwill of farmers to make their living and farmers wanted no government interference in their business. Surprisingly, the medical establishment in England also defended the position of inaction because they believed that it was unnecessary to take special precautions where tuberculous milk was concerned. In 1913, an order was handed down that required dairy farmers to keep milk from tuberculous and nontuberculous cows separate from each other, but no measures were put in place to prevent farmers from selling both. By 1914, in many of the bigger cities and wealthier suburbs in Britain, it was possible to buy milk that was certified to be nontuberculous, but it was more expensive so its sale and consumption were limited.

The outbreak of World War I pushed the fight for bovine TB control measures to the back burner in Britain. Even in wartime when supplies of milk were scarce, pasteurization was not supported in spite of the fact that it both improved the safety of milk and increased its storage life. Concerns about pasteurizing milk included the notion that it would reduce the social standing of veterinarians, promote tooth decay, diminish the incentive to produce clean milk, and reduce the nutritional value of milk. In the late 1920s, it was reported that bovine TB accounted for nearly half all TB-related lymph node and skin diseases, and about a third of other nonpulmonary forms of TB.

In the end, prevention efforts had very little to do with the events that finally stemmed the tide of bovine TB in Britain. Because TB is a disease that is dependent on social conditions, it is no surprise that changes in society finally influenced the decline of bovine TB in Britain. First, a deepening economic depression in the 1930s reduced milk consumption among the poorest children of Britain, which by extension reduced the occurrence of milk-borne TB. Additionally, between World War I and World War II there was a huge increase in the use of powdered milk because it was cheap, could be stored, had guaranteed nutritional value, and was almost sterile. In response to decreasing demand for their product, fresh milk producers finally adopted pasteurization so that milk would have a 24-hour shelf life. However, pasteurization standards were not in place in Britain until after World War II and in 1946, 7 percent to 10 percent of the pasteurized milk sold in London still contained live TB bacteria (Dormandy, 2001). If bovine TB prevention measures, including TB skin testing for cows and pasteurization of milk, had been adopted in a timely manner a great deal of sickness and death could have been avoided in Britain.

An Austrian physician, Clemens Freiherr Baron von Pirquet (1874–1929), was the first to use tuberculin skin testing in humans. By 1907, he had observed several important characteristics of TB skin test reactions. First, he noticed that it took one or two days for a reaction to the skin test to occur. Second, since many children without obvious signs of TB had a positive reaction to the skin test, Pirquet deduced that they had latent TB and that this form of the disease was compatible with overall good health. If contact with tuberculin produced no reaction, he determined that there had been no prior exposure to TB. Through these observations, Pirquet demonstrated that a simple skin test for humans could identify the important differences among TB infection, TB disease, and no TB exposure. As TB skin testing became more widely used, some reactions, both positive and negative, were determined to be false but the overall value of the test far outweighed the difficulties. By the time of Pirquet's death in the late 1920s, TB skin testing was common.

EARLY TREATMENTS AND CURES

Early treatment of TB was bound by the lack of medical and scientific knowledge, and efforts to cure the disease often added to a patient's suffering instead of bringing relief. Before the real cause of TB was discovered, people believed that the development of consumption was related to an inborn, familial predisposition toward the disease. This perception appeared to be supported by the frequent occurrence of multiple cases of TB within the same family, but the discovery of *M. tuberculosis* would eventually tell the real tale. Even after the biological cause of TB was known, it would still be many years before the first really effective treatments were discovered. From ancient times until the discovery of an antibiotic that could kill TB bacteria, early treatment regimens and "cures" were every bit as misinformed and futile as the first assumptions about the cause of TB.

From antiquity up to the mid-19th century, bloodletting was a popular medical practice that was used to treat a variety of illnesses, including TB. Bloodletting was practiced in conjunction with the contemporary theory of disease, with practitioners working to release evil spirits, exorcise demons, or release toxins and impurities depending on the historical era in question. Draining one to four pints of blood through multiple incisions over large areas of the body was typical. When the patient became faint, the treatment was stopped. As the practice of bleeding diminished over time, other medical practices that were equally horrific to patients with TB flourished. Blood cupping was a method used to draw infection from tuberculous lesions. It was practiced in several countries for many years after bloodletting was abandoned. During cupping, a small incision was made in the skin over an area of suspected TB infection and a heated glass cup was placed on the site. As the glass of the cup and the air within it cooled and contracted, blood, tissue fluid, and infectious material were sucked out through the incision in the hope that the cause of TB was being released from the body along with the other substances that were extracted.

Tuberculous skin lesions were attacked with a variety of infusions, ointments, potions, lotions, inhalations, and salves. In the 1840s, iodine solution that was administered by mouth, rubbed into the skin, mixed with food, added to bath water, or given in combination with mercury pills became a popular TB treatment. Although it was noted that some doses of iodine, especially when it was combined with mercury, caused serious nervous system damage, the benefit to the patient was still considered to outweigh the shortcomings of the treatment. Less dangerous and less expensive by far, cod-liver oil gained favor as a TB treatment

---

The Barber Pole

From 1100 to 1500, the church forbade priests to perform bloodletting and educated physicians avoided performing surgery because it was not considered a respectable medical pursuit. As a result, the practice of bloodletting was left to the barbers— the professionals who lanced veins and abscesses, and performed amputations of arms and legs during these years. A red-and-white striped pole was used to advertise the shops of barber-surgeons who did bloodletting as well as haircuts. The pole represents the stick that a patient would hold onto while being bled, the white stripes represent the bandages, and the red stripes represent the blood. The traditional red and white barber pole still greets patrons at many barbershops today even though the services offered are now limited to grooming.

---

in the 1850s. In all enlightened countries, cod-liver oil became the primary agent of cure for the sick and it was consistently used as an additional remedy to any treatment given for TB.

Frauds and great intellects alike contributed to the vast array of worthless, dangerous, or occasionally gruesome remedies offered up for the cure of TB. But even during these bleak decades of medical darkness, one treatment actually offered relief to a multitude of people with TB. Laudanum, an opium-based narcotic, was a miraculous elixir that eased the suffering of many with its pain-killing and highly sedating effects. In spite of the fact that laudanum contained morphine, the fear of becoming addicted was not a concern for those suffering with symptoms of advanced TB. Though its quality and price varied, the comforting properties of laudanum were undisputed and it was the most widely used therapeutic standby of its day.

THE SANATORIUM CURE

Throughout the centuries, belief in a fresh air cure for TB was continuously popular. Open-air sea voyages and retreats to the countryside were often all a doctor had to offer an ailing TB patient. By the late 18th century, it was well recognized that sometimes TB patients stopped getting worse and some even got better during the natural course of the disease. Early ideas about innate resistance to the progression of TB and the curative power of fresh air, exercise, and wholesome food became the basis of a therapeutic approach that would become the foundation of TB treatment for nearly a hundred years—the sanatorium cure. The first facility specifically devoted to the treatment of lung diseases was opened in Germany in 1859 by Dr. Hermann Brehmer. More like a spa than a hospital,

Dr. Brehmer's institution served a wealthy clientele with a prescribed regimen of diet, fresh air, and exercise.

In America, TB sanatoriums (variously referred to as sanitariums) were more like hospitals than spas, providing care to patients who were chronically ill with TB. Although facilities differed greatly from one to another, the concept of the sanatorium cure was based on two principles. First, even though the practice of medicine could do little on its own to treat TB, it could intervene in the course of the disease by capitalizing on the curative powers of nature, rest, fresh air, and exercise. Second, even though recuperation was believed to be the product of the patient's own vigorous defense against TB, the benefits of rest and exercise could only be achieved under medical supervision.

The ever-increasing influx of young, often poor, immigrants to America multiplied the already immense burden of TB. Additionally, because of the dread of contagion, Americans began to place increased emphasis on hygiene and cleanliness in the belief that the immune system was strengthened by improved social,

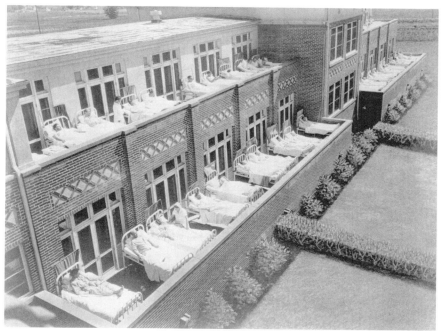

Tuberculosis patients lie in beds on the porch of the Jewish Consumptive Relief Society sanatorium, in Lakewood, Colorado (circa 1920). Fresh air, rest, good nutrition, and medical supervision were the basic elements of the sanatorium cure for TB. Courtesy of the Denver Public Library, Western History Collection, Call Number X-28623.

sanitary, and nutritional conditions. As increased measures of disease control became necessary, placing TB patients under the strict supervision of a doctor became the standard of care in America. Fear of infection and the appeal of a cure were in large part responsible for the rapid expansion of the sanatorium movement, but social and economic factors also determined how patients with TB were treated in the United States.

In 1884, Edward Livingston Trudeau established the first sanatorium in the United States. The Adirondack Cottage Sanitarium in Saranac Lake, New York, began as an experiment for Trudeau who set out to prove that the fate of patients with TB was dependent both on how they lived and on medical supervision. In an effort to fill the beds of his sanatorium and to prove his theory of TB recovery, Trudeau opened his facility as a charitable institution to serve poor TB patients who did not have the ability to care for themselves.

The treatment regimen at Saranac included an outdoor life, a special diet, close patient monitoring by physicians, and hygiene practices designed to control the spread of infection. To monitor the results of his experiment, Trudeau collected data from former patients who had been discharged from the sanitarium. Since many sanitarium-treated patients described themselves as well at the time of follow-up, Trudeau concluded that early diagnosis and immediate sanatorium treatment could result in a TB cure. Consequently, future sanatoria in the United States followed the Saranac method, although specific admissions policies, diet, and exercise regimens often depended on the social agency or physician in charge of the facility.

Even though the sanatorium cure in America was established as a charitable movement, the price of charity was often high for the poor patients who were served. A rigid standard of behavior was often imposed on the patients and small fees were sometimes charged as a way to attract the "most desirable" poor people, leaving the free facilities to treat the most chronic, debilitated patients. Authorities believed that combating contagion depended on confining ill patients and an extraordinary degree of control was imposed on poor people who had TB. In some facilities, a work cure was substituted for a rest cure so that poor invalids were not encouraged to become healthy slackers. Wealthy patients sought the sanatorium

---

Contagion and the Sanatorium Cure

When TB was identified as an infectious disease, the sanatorium movement quickly expanded in America. In 1900, there were only 34 sanatoria, with 4,485 beds, in the United States. By 1925, 536 sanatoria, with 673,338 beds, were in operation throughout the country (Rothman, 1995).

cure too, but the rich segregated themselves from the poor and created their own society among the dying.

The sanatorium cure formed the foundation of TB treatment for at least a hundred years. Sanatoriums persisted through the discovery of the cause of TB and the social changes of two world wars, but did the cure work? An evaluation of records from 564 patients treated in New York sanatoria between 1938 and 1948 found that the outcome of sanatorium treatment was mostly dependent on one factor—how sick the patient was when he or she entered the sanatorium. For patients with minimal disease, follow-up at both 5- and 15-year intervals after their stay in the sanatorium showed that the majority still had inactive TB; 13 percent had died of TB by the 15-year follow-up. However, the outlook for patients who entered the sanatorium with advanced TB was much worse—half of these patients died within two years and 60 percent were dead by the five-year follow-up. Only 22 percent of patients with the most advanced TB experienced remission as a result of the sanatorium cure, a dismal prognosis indeed (Daniel, 1997).

The sanatorium movement represented a massive effort to care for the victims of TB; unfortunately, improved diet, fresh air, exercise, and rest were inadequate measures for many patients and TB remained the serial killer it had always been. While the world waited for the breakthrough discovery that would bring a cure, the fight against TB embraced additional methods of treatment and renewed prevention efforts.

SURGICAL INTERVENTION

Rest was a well-accepted rule of TB therapy, as demonstrated by the central role it played in most sanatorium regimens. However, even if a patient spent the majority of their time reclined in a chair to partake of the fresh air, the lungs themselves still had to work to breathe. The early observation that TB improved in a few patients following an injury that caused the lung to collapse made doctors consider the idea of surgically inducing lung collapse to produce a cure for TB.

Carlo Forliani is considered the pioneer of surgically induced collapse of the lung, or artificial pneumothorax as it is called, for the treatment of TB. After experimenting on animals to develop procedures to cause the lung on one side to collapse, Forliani became convinced that the same procedure could be safely done in humans. In 1894, Forliani performed the procedure on a 15-year-old patient with advanced TB. She tolerated the surgery well and within months Forliani noted that her condition had improved. The procedure was adopted as a treatment for TB in both Europe and the United States. The development of improved x-ray diagnostics in the early 20th century greatly enhanced a doctor's ability to predict which patients would most likely benefit from artificial pneumothorax.

Over the next 25 years, artificial pneumothorax was used to treat more than 100,000 patients with TB, and although the benefit of the procedure was described by many, no study of the actual outcome of the treatment was ever conducted. Because medical practitioners were so convinced of the benefit of lung collapse to treat TB, alternative surgical procedures were introduced and more extensive surgical interventions were pioneered.

Although artificial pneumothorax and a few surgical procedures undoubtedly helped some patients with TB, the treatment was not without risks, including loss of lung function, increased burden on the patient's heart, and physical disfigurement. In spite of the precarious balance between the benefit and risks associated with artificial pneumothorax, by the 1920s most sanatorium patients were clamoring for the procedure. The combination of surgical intervention and the sanatorium cure ushered in an era where active TB treatment was balanced with the time-worn principle of rest.

PREVENTION: THE BACILLUS CALMETTE-GUÉRIN VACCINE

In 1900, Léon Charles Albert Calmette and Camille Guérin of France began to work on producing a vaccine to protect against TB infection. Using a weak strain of tubercle bacilli that they developed from infected cows, Calmette and Guérin began experiments in which they inoculated animals to try to induce immunity to TB without causing the disease. Working in secret throughout World War I, they vaccinated several kinds of animals and then deliberately exposed them to TB to see if the vaccine prevented the infection. By the end of the war, Calmette and Guérin were convinced that their vaccine was safe and that it was effective in preventing TB in animals. Most importantly, they believed it would work in humans as well as it did in animals.

Human testing was approached with great caution. To determine if the vaccine was effective, it needed to be given to someone who was not already infected with TB. For ethical reasons, however, the vaccine also needed to be administered to someone who was at very high risk of dying from TB. On July 18, 1921, the Bacillus Calmette-Guérin (BCG) vaccine was administered to a human being for the first time. The first patient to receive the TB vaccine was a newborn baby whose mother had died of TB a few hours after giving birth. The baby was at very high risk of contracting the infection and for this reason, it was determined that he would be a good candidate for the vaccine test. The first vaccine test was a success—the inoculated baby showed no ill effects from the vaccine and he was subsequently raised in good health, free from TB.

From the beginning, the BCG vaccination and its creators were not without critics. Calmette was accused of using fuzzy statistics to support his research.

Political wrangling between countries and skepticism tempered the eagerness to accept Calmette's claims of success. In spite of international squabbling, more than 100,000 doses of vaccine were given to infants without any known serious complications from 1924 to 1928. Under pressure from the French government, in 1928, the League of Nations, an intergovernmental organization founded after World War I to settle disputes though diplomacy and negotiation, certified that BCG was safe for use in humans. In 1929, Calmette reported that the death rate from TB was 33 percent for unvaccinated children compared with 4 percent for vaccinated children with similar exposure (Daniel, 1997).

Germany was one of the countries that embraced the BCG vaccine with enthusiasm. Between February and April 1930, the Municipal Children's Hospital in Lübeck administered an oral BCG vaccination to 249 babies within the first 10 days of their lives. In April, an unforeseen tragedy began to unfold when babies that had been vaccinated with BCG in February began to die from devastating cases of TB. Despite frenzied efforts to save them, 67 babies had died by June and another 80 were seriously ill. The exact number of babies that eventually died and the exact reason that they did will never be fully known—on April 30 the German government silenced all further official information regarding the situation.

By May, a full cover-up of what had really happened was under way, and official hospital records and existing vaccine supplies were destroyed. It had already come to light, and could not later be denied, that some members of the hospital staff had been engaged in their own research with virulent human TB bacteria. Opponents of the vaccine were quick to say that their predictions of disaster had been correct. Vaccine advocates from both France and Germany were eager to learn what had really happened. An official inquiry by the German government was undertaken and, in spite of the recent tragedy, investigation quickly validated that the BCG vaccine was safe. So, what happened to the vaccinated babies who died in Lübeck? In the end, it was determined that the dreadful events were the result of blatant disregard of established hospital safety precautions. Highly virulent TB cultures that were intended for research purposes had either inadvertently contaminated the vaccine supply or had actually been administered to the babies by mistake. After this debacle, the future of the vaccine was in serious jeopardy. Several countries outright rejected its use—BCG was banned in Britain until 1947—and hostility toward it persisted in several centers in the United States and Canada for a long time.

Work and research on the BCG vaccine fortunately continued. It was subsequently determined that injection under the skin was more effective than oral administration, and it came to light that, while the vaccine offered no absolute immunity to TB, it significantly increased natural resistance to the disease. The

BCG strain was distributed to medical and academic institutions around the world so that they could establish offspring strains of the vaccine. Its administration drastically increased after World War II, and hundreds of millions of people have been immunized to date. The vaccine is safe and it is only rarely associated with side effects, such as inflammation at the vaccination site. The parent strain of bacteria from which the original vaccine was made has been lost. During the initial years of culturing the original strain to make more vaccine, the bacteria continued to lose genes, suggesting that the initial vaccine may have been much more virulent.

Studies of the BCG vaccine in different populations and in different places have shown that its effectiveness varies considerably, and its immunological mechanism, which accounts for its ability to fight TB infection, remains poorly understood. While the protective effect of the vaccine in children is widely recognized, its ability to prevent pulmonary TB in adults is more questionable and its efficacy appears to diminish over time. Today, the World Health Organization recommends BCG vaccination as early in life as possible for all infants born in areas of the world where infant TB is a problem. In the United States, the BCG vaccination has never been a part of the national campaign against TB because of its interference with skin test results and its unknown effectiveness in preventing adult TB.

PUBLIC HEALTH EFFORTS

When TB was recognized as a contagious disease, U.S. public health authorities began to regard it as their duty to protect the public from it. From 1890 to 1920, crusades against tenement housing, sweatshops, child labor, public spitting and coughing, and unpasteurized milk were mounted. Educational programs were instituted to teach the public new rules of hygiene. Mandatory reporting of TB cases to public health officials was required in many cities and TB registries were formed. Despite some positive outcomes and supposedly decent objectives, strict public health efforts to control TB had some unfortunate and unforeseen consequences. Discrimination against the sick and poor, and fear of associating with them, became commonplace because of the dread of being infected and the stigma associated with TB. For people who had TB, interstate travel was restricted, employment was sometimes denied, and forced confinement to state hospitals and public sanatoria were allowable measures used to protect the public. "Lungers need not inquire" was a sign that was commonly displayed in the windows of boardinghouses and hotels that refused to rent to people who appeared to have TB. Beginning in the 1890s and persisting through the 1930s, having TB became such a disgrace that many infected people chose to keep the disease a secret from everyone, including family and friends.

Since TB was seen as a disease of the poor, charity became a large part of the effort to control it. Associations were formed and public participation in events to raise money to combat it became fashionable. The National Association for the Study and Prevention of Tuberculosis, the first nationwide voluntary health organization focused on conquering one specific disease, was founded in 1904. A few years later, a doctor working at a small sanatorium in Delaware realized that the facility was on the verge of financial ruin. He wrote a letter to his cousin Emily Bissel, who was active in the American Red Cross and had fundraising experience, and asked for her help in raising $300 to keep the sanatorium open. Having heard about a man who sold decorative stamps to fight TB in Denmark, Bissell sketched out a design and in 1907, the first American Christmas Seal was produced. She borrowed $40 to have 50,000 of them printed and sold them for a penny a piece at the local post office. Bissell became a one-woman crusader against TB, speaking at public events and working overtime to make Christmas

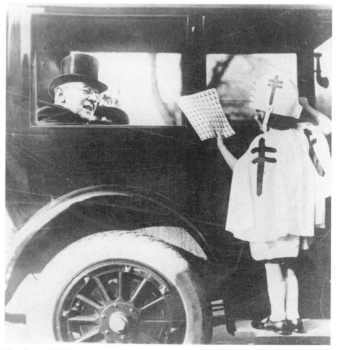

President Woodrow Wilson stops to purchase Tuberculosis Seals from a little TB crusader standing on the running board of his car in December 1923. The Christmas Seal campaign was launched in 1907 to raise money for the fight against TB. Courtesy of the Library of Congress.

Seals a success. When President Theodore Roosevelt heard about her efforts and endorsed the idea of Christmas Seals, the campaign caught on and before the Christmas season was over, she had raised over $3,000. The success of the first local Christmas stamp effort led to the adoption of the Christmas Seals program on a national level and it became a well-known feature of the holiday season, attracting enormous celebrity support and raising millions of dollars over the years in the crusade to eradicate TB.

During World War II, the need to evaluate large numbers of military recruits in a short period of time led to the development of x-ray equipment that could screen many people quickly. This technology was later put to use in mass chest x-ray screening programs that were initiated in 1947 by TB control programs across the states. Trucks and buses fitted with x-ray equipment hit the roads to root out TB in cities and towns across America. Millions of people were screened

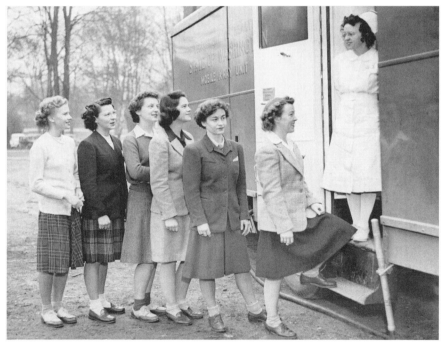

Young women lined up outside a mobile TB x-ray unit sometime in the 1940s. Trucks and buses that were specially equipped with x-ray machines screened millions of people for TB in the United States. University of Washington Libraries, Special Collections, SOC0848.

for TB in the mobile x-ray units, which became a very visible symbol of the American crusade against TB.

Public health efforts and the advent of effective antibiotic treatment tamed the TB monster in the United States. In many places in the world, however, it remains a challenge to public health and social justice, not just an infectious disease. In developing nations, TB remains a health crisis embedded in poverty and lack of access to consistent and effective treatment. TB control programs administered by international public health agencies, such as the World Health Organization, in partnership with government agencies, private foundations, corporations, and academic institutions, remain the hope of worldwide TB eradication.

5

Antibiotics: Treatment Success, Challenge, and Cure

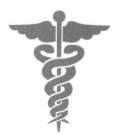

The story of antibiotics started more than 3,000 years ago when ancient people stumbled upon the discovery that some molds could be used as medicinal cures. It is not historically certain if Egyptians, Chinese, or the native peoples of Central America were the first to treat infected wounds in this manner, but it is certain that knowledge of disease at this time did not include an understanding of infectious organisms. As time went on, greater insight into the nature of disease and what could cure it was gained. In the 1860s, Louis Pasteur was the first to show that microorganisms, such as bacteria, caused many diseases. Later on, he discovered that one type of bacteria could prevent the growth of or kill another type of bacteria, although he didn't know that the reason was that the bacteria were producing an antibiotic.

The term "antibiotic" was first used in 1942 by Selman Waksman (1888–1973), the man who identified the first antibiotic that was effective against the microorganism that causes TB. Originally, antibiotics were any substance produced by a microorganism that inhibited the growth of other microorganisms. Today, antibiotics are chemically modified from original compounds found in nature (such as penicillin, which is produced by fungi) or are created by purely synthetic means.

STREPTOMYCIN: DISCOVERY OF AN ANTIBIOTIC TO FIGHT TUBERCULOSIS

Antibiotic agents like sulfonamide and penicillin had been used to fight infectious diseases for several years before a molecule that was effective against *M. tuberculosis* was discovered. Waksman, a biochemist and microbiologist, was born in the Ukraine and immigrated to the United States in 1910. After working on a family farm in New Jersey for a few years, he enrolled at Rutgers College where he began to research bacteria found in soil. These bacteria became a source of enduring interest and he studied them while he completed both his master's and doctoral degrees, eventually becoming a renowned expert in the field. In time, his attention turned from the role microorganisms played in the science of soil ecology to the concept of how drugs could treat infection.

World War II provided an incentive for research into a new area of investigation, the study of antibiotics. In the history of medicine, the discovery of

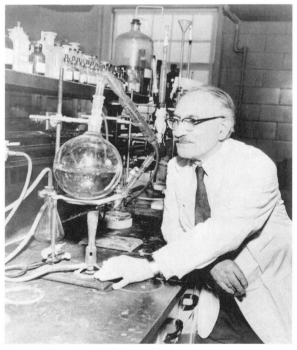

Dr. Selman Waksman, the microbiologist who discovered streptomycin, at work in the laboratory in 1953. Courtesy of the Library of Congress.

antibiotics is one of the greatest accomplishments in the fight against disease. Using his background in soil microbiology, Waksman assumed a lead role in the investigation of antibiotics and in 1940, he and his team of scientists at Rutgers isolated an antibiotic that effectively inhibited the growth of TB bacteria. Initial excitement dimmed when the antibiotic proved to be too toxic to use in humans or animals, but anticipation began to build with the hope that a breakthrough was near.

The first real progress toward a cure for TB came in 1943 when a poultry pathologist sent a culture of an organism he had found in throat of a sick chicken to Waksman and his team. After a few months of work, two graduate students in Waksman's lab identified the organism as *Streptomyces griseus*, a soil organism that had originally been identified by Waksman in 1919. From this strain, they isolated a new antibiotic, which they named streptomycin. They tested its activity against 22 different bacteria and found that it had robust activity against several microorganisms, including some that were immune to the effects of penicillin. M. *tuberculosis* was among the microorganisms that streptomycin was active against and in laboratory studies, it had lower toxicity in animals than other previously isolated antibiotics. A new era in the fight against TB had begun.

H. Corwin Hinshaw and William Feldman, two scientists from the Mayo Clinic in Rochester, Minnesota, heard about the discovery of streptomycin and visited Waksman's lab. Although Hinshaw and Feldman had no experience with antibiotics, they were eager students of TB. Waksman sent them a supply of crude streptomycin that contained less than 6 percent of the active drug and the first studies of the new antibiotic began. Eight guinea pigs infected with TB became the subjects of experimentation—four were treated with streptomycin and four were left untreated so that they could be used for comparison. Hinshaw and Feldman injected the infected guinea pigs with streptomycin every three hours around the clock for six weeks. When the first experiment was completed in June 1944, all four guinea pigs that had not received streptomycin had more advanced TB infection and two of them had died. Of the guinea pigs that had been treated with streptomycin, all four lived and their TB infections had disappeared. Additional animal experiments were conducted and the results were the same. Hinshaw and Feldman were convinced—streptomycin cured TB in guinea pigs.

On November 20, 1944, the first dose of streptomycin was administered to a human patient who was critically ill with TB. Although history has documented her only as Patricia T., she was a 21-year-old woman who had been a patient in a sanatorium for a year. Her illness had worsened in spite of sanatorium care and her doctor was certain that she would die if the disease was allowed to advance without intervention. Her physician consulted Hinshaw, and the doctors recognized an opportunity to test streptomycin in a human and, if all went well, to help a dying patient. Together, they approached the young woman with their novel treatment plan and she agreed to become, in essence, a human guinea pig by beginning treatment with streptomycin. Using the same supply of drug that was used in the animal experiments, Patricia T. was injected with streptomycin every three hours. The injections were painful and produced some unpleasant side effects including pain, fever, and headache. After 10 days of treatment, Patricia T. needed time to recover from the severe reactions to the treatment and the injections were stopped. A month later, streptomycin injections were restarted for another 10-day period. With great anticipation, the first post-streptomycin chest x-ray was taken to determine if the treatment had produced any change in Patricia T.'s condition. Much to the disappointment of doctors and patient alike, the first x-ray after treatment showed no change from her pre-streptomycin condition.

In January 1945, a more purified form of streptomycin became available. Patricia T. agreed to start treatment again and she began to receive daily streptomycin in doses that would subsequently become the standard of treatment. This course of streptomycin continued for 45 days, and as time went on, the hope for success began to be realized—Patricia T. started to get better. The number of bacteria in her sputum began to decrease and some of the disease in her lungs disappeared completely. Treatment with streptomycin cured TB in Patricia T., and for the first time in history, doctors had a real way to fight the dreaded disease. After a period of recovery, Patricia T. eventually married and had three children. A follow-up examination in August 1954 determined that her TB had remained inactive since her treatment with streptomycin. The discovery of streptomycin was considered a scientific breakthrough of epic proportion, and as a result, Selman Waksman was awarded several international honors, including the Nobel Prize in Medicine in 1952. After centuries of medical defenselessness and hopeful guesswork, TB was no longer a disease without a cure.

MORE ANTIBIOTICS TO TREAT TUBERCULOSIS

Almost immediately after streptomycin was introduced to treat TB, the phenomenon of treatment resistance emerged. In response to treatment with a single antibiotic, the bacteria quickly evolved and streptomycin alone proved to be no match for new strains of M. *tuberculosis*. The development of other anti-TB drugs quickly followed the discovery of streptomycin, and it became apparent that treatment resistance could be overcome if more than one drug was used at a time. Combination therapy with multiple antibiotics became standard treatment and it remains so today.

To be an effective anti-TB drug, an antibiotic must have antibacterial activity, the capacity to inhibit the development of resistance, and the ability to kill the living microorganisms that remain inside the cells. If TB bacteria become resistant to an antibiotic, drug-resistant strains of TB that are harder to treat develop. To prevent this, an effective treatment regimen must include multiple drugs that can kill the bacteria. When two or more drugs are used at the same time, each one helps prevent the bacteria from becoming resistant to the other drugs. Until the introduction of the antibiotic rifampin in the 1963, TB treatment for a one- to two-year period of time was required to prevent recurrence. Rifampin allowed the initiation of what is referred to as short-course treatment, which means that fewer than 12 months of antibiotic treatment is now sufficient to treat TB.

Since it is usually not known which two antibiotics will be effective in any specific case, four first-line antibiotics are usually prescribed to treat TB: isoniazid, rifampin, pyrazinamide, and ethambutal. When these four drugs are used at the beginning of therapy, 95 percent of patients will respond to at least two of them, and treatment is very effective as long as patients take all the drugs as often and for as long as they were prescribed. The usual duration of antibiotic treatment with this regimen of drugs is six to nine months, but improvement in a patient's condition occurs rapidly and TB quickly becomes less infectious. Over the months, specific milestones are used to determine if treatment has been a success or failure. When there is concern that treatment is not working, a doctor evaluates the need to change antibiotics, investigates the bacteria to determine if it is resistant to specific anti-TB drugs, and makes sure that the patient is taking their medicine exactly as it was prescribed. Treatment failure usually occurs

---

TB Treatment Milestones

After one or two months of treatment, most patients will:
- Have no fever
- Be feeling well
- Regain lost weight
- Have a negative smear culture

After three months of treatment:
- There is concern about treatment failure if the sputum culture remains positive

After five to six months of treatment:
- A positive smear indicates that the treatment has failed

Treatment success is certain when:
- A sputum specimen is negative for M. *tuberculosis*

because a patient is not taking their medicine correctly or the treatment that was prescribed is not adequate.

Standard short-course TB treatment is divided into two phases. In the initial phase, the majority of the bacteria are killed, symptoms get better, and patients become noncontagious. Because TB bacteria die very slowly, treatment is continued to make sure that any leftover bacteria are killed so that the patient does not relapse, meaning that they do not get sick again after treatment is stopped. Even though patients feel better after being treated for a short time, it takes at least six months for antibiotics to kill all the TB bacteria and it is very important that patients continue to take antibiotics regularly for as long as necessary to ensure that TB has been cured. Additionally, when leftover bacteria are allowed to survive, they may become resistant to the drugs they have already been exposed to, making future treatment more difficult and costly.

Treating patients with TB and HIV co-infection is more complex and requires expertise in the management of both diseases. Treatment recommendations for TB in adults with HIV co-infection are basically the same as those for patients who do not have HIV with a few important exceptions. The development of rifampin resistance or relapse has been noted among HIV-infected patients who have advanced immune system suppression. This requires more frequent dosing of antibiotics in the continuation phase of treatment than what may otherwise be recommended. Strategies that promote adherence to TB treatment are especially important for patients with HIV-related TB. Treatment adherence means that a patient takes their medication exactly as it is prescribed for as long as it is necessary. Because HIV-infected patients are often taking numerous medications, special care must also be taken to ensure that other medications don't interact with anti-TB medications. Of particular concern is the interaction of the rifamycin group of antibiotics (including rifampin) with antiretroviral agents, the drugs that are the mainstay of HIV/AIDS treatment.

The basic principles that underpin the treatment of pulmonary TB also apply to extra-pulmonary forms of the disease. Although relatively few studies have examined treatment of extra-pulmonary TB, increasing evidence suggests that 6- to 9-month regimens that include isoniazid and rifampin are effective. Thus, a 6-month course of therapy is recommended for treating TB involving any site except the central nervous system, for which a 9- to 12-month regimen is recommended. Additionally, more prolonged treatment should also be considered for patients with TB that is slow to respond regardless of where in the body it occurs.

STRATEGIES FOR IMPROVING TREATMENT ADHERENCE

Complete TB treatment requires that a combination of antibiotic drugs be taken for a long period of time. When patients are not treated correctly, they can remain sick for a longer time and continue to be contagious, or they can get better for a while and relapse, becoming contagious all over again. Improperly treated patients are likely to develop strains of TB that are not responsive to the first-line antibiotics, which makes curing individual cases more complicated and adds to the overall burden of disease in the world. In spite of all the problems that are caused by inadequate or incorrect TB treatment, it is very difficult for many patients to take several medications for a long time. Factors like poverty, inability to pay for medications, social stigma, and lack of long-term access to treatment affect the ability of many patients to fully complete their treatment.

The directly observed therapy, short-course (DOTS) program is a treatment adherence plan to ensure worldwide access to antibiotic agents and trained medical personnel. The plan was launched by the World Health Organization in the early 1990s with the immediate goal of improving TB treatment and the ultimate goal of eliminating global TB once and for all. Applied with great success around the world, the principles of the DOTS program comprise: (1) a political commitment from all countries that includes increased and sustained financing for TB treatment; (2) detection of TB cases through quality-assured laboratory diagnosis; (3) standardized treatment with supervised drug administration and patient support; (4) an effective drug supply and management system; and (5) a monitoring and evaluation system that includes reports on treatment outcomes. The early success of DOTS was demonstrated when, in 2003, the World Health Organization reported that more than 10 million TB patients had been successfully treated, with more than 90 percent of the successes reported in patients who lived in developing countries where the disease causes the most suffering, economic loss, and death.

One of the keys to the success of the DOTS program lies in the supervision of treatment to ensure that patients take all their medicine for the right amount of time. Sometimes treatment supervision means that a health care worker actually watches a patient take their medication every day. This practice helps make sure that patients take their antibiotics regularly and correctly, and it gives health care providers the opportunity to deliver appropriate care and support. Depending on the local conditions, treatment supervision may take place at a health facility, in the workplace, in the community, or at home. Sometimes incentives, small rewards that encourage or motivate, are used to encourage patients to continue and complete treatment. Food, travel vouchers, grocery store vouchers, nutritional supplements, or money are used to encourage patients to continue to take their medicine for as long as necessary. Additionally, free transportation, reminder letters or phone calls, and other assistance help patients keep appointments and complete their treatment.

With the potential to cure 9 out of 10 cases of TB, the DOTS strategy is considered to be a very effective health intervention program. In spite of the fact that many countries have adopted it, the spread of TB continues to outpace the reach of DOTS. The inability to expand the program as rapidly as needed has been blamed on factors such as a lack of political commitment, insufficient financial resources, inadequate health system organizations and personnel in developing countries, and insufficient drug supplies.

Other strategies to maximize the likelihood that patients will adhere to treatment include collaboration between local health departments and community-based organizations that can provide case management to ensure a continuity of services. Clear education and instruction about medication and potential side effects should be provided to patients in their native language. If possible, it is helpful for health care professionals to seek the involvement of family members when they provide TB education and treatment instruction to a patient so that support and encouragement are available during the long course of treatment.

TREATMENT OF DRUG-RESISTANT TUBERCULOSIS

Drug-resistant TB can occur when someone who has never had TB before becomes infected with bacteria that are already resistant to first-line anti-TB drugs or when someone has received an inadequate course of TB treatment. Incorrect or incomplete TB treatment allows the live bacteria that are left behind to adjust to the first-line anti-TB drugs and they become ineffective. Patients with multidrug-resistant TB can be resistant to one or several first-line treatments. Multidrug-resistant TB is more difficult to treat and requires the combination of several second-line anti-TB drugs for 18 to 24 months and at least 9 months after a sputum culture is negative.

Good outcomes have been achieved in treating multidrug-resistant TB with the class of antibiotics known as fluoroquinolones, a relatively new family of synthetic, broad-spectrum antibiotics. They have become a mainstay of multidrug-resistant TB treatment. Fluoroquinolones should be used with some restraint for the treatment of non-TB illnesses since the development of bacteria that are resistant to this class of antibiotics would severely compromise treatment of multidrug-resistant TB. Because these drugs work across a wide range of illnesses, they are frequently used haphazardly in situations where other antibiotics would work just as well. This exposes more bacteria to the fluoroquinolones, increasing the chances that drug-resistant strains will develop. Additionally, inadequately dosed fluoroquinolones also promote the production of drug-resistant organisms. Frequent and inappropriate use of these antibiotics may create an environment that fosters the development of quinolone-resistant strains of mycobacteria, and reports of quinolone-resistant TB are becoming increasingly common.

The inclusion of second-line anti-TB drugs, like the fluoroquinolones, in DOTS programs is a very important component of multidrug-resistant TB treatment. Treating multidrug-resistant patients with first-line DOTS treatment, a regimen that used to be encouraged in developing nations, is wasteful and unnecessary because these drugs are not effective against multidrug-resistant strains. If quinolone-resistant strains of TB become widespread, the future of multidrug-resistant TB control will become even more challenging. Preventing the emergence of new antibiotic resistance is a very an important goal of multidrug-resistant TB control.

Extensively drug-resistant TB is an even more deadly and dangerous form of drug-resistant TB. Treatment success rates for cases of extensively drug-resistant TB are generally between 30 percent and 50 percent, with very poor outcomes in HIV-infected patients (LoBue, 2009). Even though extensively drug-resistant TB is still relatively rare, its global incidence is increasing and it is a serious threat to worldwide TB control. In the United States, extensively drug-resistant TB is still rare—83 cases were documented by the Centers for Disease Control and Prevention between 1993 and 2007. However, worldwide, the numbers are much larger and on the rise. For example, in the only global TB study of extensively drug-resistant TB to date, the World Health Organization reported that of multidrug-resistant TB cases in Ukraine, 15 percent were extensively drug-resistant in 2008 (Hugonnet et al., 2009).

Extensively drug-resistant forms of TB are resistant to almost all the drugs that are used to treat the disease. By definition, extensively drug-resistant TB does not respond to the two best first-line drugs (isoniazid and rifampin), any fluoroquinolone antibiotic, and at least one of three second-line injectable drugs. In some cases, extensively drug-resistant TB can be treated and cured but a successful outcome depends on the extent of drug resistance, the severity of the disease, whether the patient's immune system is weakened, and how well the patient follows the treatment regimen. Treatment failures and subsequent deaths are more common among patients with extensively drug-resistant TB, and the drugs available to treat it are associated with serious side effects.

TREATMENT OF LATENT TUBERCULOSIS

Treatment of latent TB infection is essential to controlling and eliminating TB in the United States. Treatment of latent TB substantially reduces the risk that infection will progress to disease. If a person has a positive tuberculin skin test or TB blood test, and the presence of active TB infection is ruled out, the relative benefits of treating the latent infection will be assessed on the basis of individual patient circumstances. Factors that are considered include the risk of developing

TB disease, the level of commitment regarding treatment completion, and access to resources that are available to ensure treatment adherence. When a person has a positive reaction to a TB skin test, a red swollen area appears at the site of the injection 48 to 72 hours after the test. The size of the swelling that occurs and the individual risk factors for developing active TB are evaluated together to help determine the need for treatment.

The potential success of treatment for latent TB infection often depends on a good understanding of the risks and benefits of treatment. A person considering treatment for latent TB infection must understand that as long as TB germs are present in the body, they can begin to multiply and cause disease. Individuals who are at especially high risk of latent TB progression to active disease include people with recent TB infection, people with certain medical conditions such as HIV, and people who are taking medication that may alter the immune system's ability to fight TB. Unlike TB disease, which initially requires treatment with four drugs, latent TB infection is treated with one medication. Completing treatment for latent TB can reduce the risk of developing active TB disease by 90 percent. Certain groups, including the homeless, the elderly, substance abusers, people who are foreign-born, and migrant workers, present unique challenges during latent TB treatment and they have needs that require special consideration.

Treatment adherence for people with latent TB may be particularly difficult because they are not sick or contagious, and because treatment is long and may be associated with some side effects. Because taking prescribed anti-TB drugs exactly as prescribed for as long as they are prescribed is such an important element of TB treatment, barriers to good treatment adherence need to be addressed. Potential factors that can compromise good treatment adherence include misinformation about TB, personal beliefs about health and health care practices, drug side effects, drug interactions, limited financial resources, co-existing medical conditions, language barriers, and real or perceived stigma related to TB.

The three recommended treatment regimens for latent TB use isoniazid or rifampin in different doses and for different lengths of time, depending on the specific plan. The preferred treatment regimen uses isoniazid either once or twice daily for a period of nine months. If the person who is being treated for latent TB is in contact with someone who has isoniazid- or multidrug-resistant TB, the typical treatment regimen is modified to ensure success. If latent TB has occurred as the result of exposure to and infection from a person with multidrug-resistant TB or extensively drug-resistant TB, preventive treatment may not be an option. Doctor visits should occur on a monthly basis during treatment for latent TB to assess adherence and identify any potential side effects.

Who Should Be Treated for Latent Tuberculosis?

People in these high-risk groups should be given treatment for latent TB if the size of the swelling on their forearm in reaction to a Mantoux tuberculin skin test measures bigger than 5 millimeters:

- People who have HIV
- People who have had recent contact with someone who has TB
- People with findings on a chest x-ray that are consistent with old TB
- Patients who have had organ transplants because antirejection drugs suppress the immune system
- People who have suppressed immune systems for other reasons

In addition, people in these high-risk groups should be considered for treatment of latent TB if the size of the swelling on their forearm in reaction to a Mantoux tuberculin skin test measures bigger than 10 millimeters:

- People who recently arrived in the United States from countries with high TB prevalence
- I.V. drug users
- Residents and employees of high-risk settings (e.g., correctional facilities, nursing homes, homeless shelters, hospitals and other health care facilities)
- Mycobacteriology laboratory personnel
- Persons with clinical conditions that make them high-risk
- Children under four years of age, or children and adolescents exposed to adults in high-risk categories

SIDE EFFECTS OF TUBERCULOSIS TREATMENT

Side effects, especially gastrointestinal upset, are relatively common in the first few weeks of anti-TB therapy. Because of the importance of completing treatment, however, first-line anti-TB drugs, particularly rifampin, must not be discontinued because of minor side effects. Although taking anti-TB drugs with food delays or moderately decreases the absorption of the drugs, the effects of food on the drugs are not considered to be very important. Thus, if patients have minor stomach upset or nausea because of the first-line drugs, taking them with meals or changing the time they are taken may be recommended. To achieve the best treatment effect, taking the medication with food is preferable to splitting a dose or changing to a second-line drug. Other potential side effects that are associated with anti-TB medications and that should be reported to the health

Anti-TB Drug Side Effects

The drugs used to treat TB are relatively safe, but sometimes they may cause side effects. Some side effects are not considered serious, and continuing treatment in spite of them is very important. Other side effects are more serious and patients should immediately call a health care provider if they experience any of them. It may be necessary to stop taking the medication or to return to the clinic for tests.

These symptoms are considered serious side effects of anti-TB medications:
- No appetite
- Nausea
- Vomiting
- Yellowish skin or eyes
- Fever for three days or longer
- Abdominal pain
- Tingling fingers or toes
- Skin rash
- Easy bleeding and/or bruising
- Aching joints
- Dizziness
- Tingling or numbness around the mouth
- Blurred or changed vision
- Ringing in the ears and/or hearing loss

These symptoms are not considered serious side effects of anti-TB medications:
- Rifampin can turn urine, saliva, or tears an orange color (patients may be advised not to wear soft contact lenses because they may get stained)
- Rifampin can cause sensitivity to the sun (patients should use a good sunscreen and cover exposed areas)
- Rifampin makes birth control pills less effective (women patients who take rifampin should use another form of birth control)

care provider include unexplained weight loss, nausea or vomiting, persistent numbness in the hands or feet, persistent weakness, fatigue, fever, abdominal tenderness, and easy bruising or bleeding.

The most serious common side effect associated with taking anti-TB drugs is hepatitis. Hepatitis is injury to the liver that impairs its normal functions, including detoxification of the system, regulation of blood composition, and production of bile to help digestion. If hepatitis occurs, isoniazid, pyrazinamide, and rifampin, all of which are potential causes of liver injury, should be stopped immediately. Blood tests are performed and questions are asked about exposure to other substances that may be toxic to the liver, especially alcohol. Two or more anti-TB medications that are not toxic to the liver, such as ethambutal or a fluoroquinolone, may be used until the cause of the hepatitis is identified. When hepatitis resolves and symptoms have significantly improved, the first-line medications are restarted one at a time. Close monitoring and review of symptoms, along with repeated blood tests to measure liver function, are used to take care of patients with hepatitis.

Medications that a patient may be taking for another medical condition may interact with anti-TB medications. To avoid drug interactions, doctors should be aware of all medications patients are taking. For woman of childbearing age, it is important to note that rifampin may decrease the blood levels of oral contraceptives, which makes them less effective; patients being treated with anti-TB drugs should discuss methods of birth control with their health care provider. Also of note, rifampin is contraindicated in HIV-infected individuals who are being treated with certain antiretroviral agents.

6

Tuberculosis in the Arts: From the Ancients to *Moulin Rouge!*

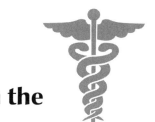

T he social environment influences the likelihood of developing TB, and in turn, TB goes on to influence the society in which it develops. No-where has this been more obvious than in the arts, where the notori-ous impact of TB has affected many different artistic genres, including painting, literature, music, and film. TB is a disease whose very history is better informed because of the contributions of numerous artists who suffered from it and used it thematically in their work. The disease and its influence on society have been represented through various forms of artistic expression from prehistoric Egyptian art, to 18th-century novels and poems, to contemporary big-screen movies. Art has helped to define the perception of TB and the disease has helped to define the art of various historical periods.

TUBERCULOSIS AND LITERATURE

Across the centuries, the writers and poets who suffered from or died of TB have chronicled its history. The influence TB had on their artistic works and the subsequent effect their poetry and prose had on society are inestimable. TB killed some prominent writers and caused untold suffering for others; their work leaves no doubt that the disease influenced their perceptions and their literature.

Some Prominent Writers Affected by TB across the Generations

Poet John Keats (1795–1821); American author Washington Irving (1783–1859); the Brontë sisters (1800s); American poet Ralph Waldo Emerson (1803–1882); poet Elizabeth Barrett Browning (1806–1861); Henry David Thoreau (1817–1862); Robert Louis Stevenson (1850–1894); Russian playwright Anton Chekhov (1860–1904); novelist Franz Kafka (1883–1924); America's premier playwright Eugene O'Neill (1888–1953); American detective novelist Dashiell Hammett (1894–1961); Thomas Wolfe (1900–1938); George Orwell (1903–1950); French author, philosopher, and journalist Albert Camus (1913–1960); poet Dylan Thomas (1914–1953); and American author and poet Charles Bukowski (1920–1994).

Since travel to a place with a more agreeable climate was frequently the best medicine a doctor had to offer a TB patient in the 1800s, it is not surprising that the Scottish-born writer Robert Louis Stevenson (1850–1894) spent much of his life on journeys in search of good health. Stevenson probably developed TB when he was a child and a chronically relapsing course of the disease plagued him throughout this life. He suffered from typical symptoms of TB such as fever, sweats, cough, and bleeding from the lungs, interspersed with periods of relative good health and literary productivity. He was 23 years old when he was diagnosed with probable "threatening phthisis" and he spent the following winter in France, the country that almost became a second home to him during the many trips he took to benefit his health. On one of his excursions there, he met an American woman named Fanny Osborne who was in the process of divorce. They fell in love and when she returned to California, Stevenson followed her. They married and when his ill health returned in 1880, the couple went to Davos, Switzerland so that Stevenson could recuperate at a treatment spa. While there, his health improved and he was allowed to write for three hours each day. He worked steadily on *Treasure Island*, the book that would subsequently bring him fame and renown as an author, and in 1882 he was well enough to return to the United Kingdom.

He had alternating periods of illness and health over the next several years, but he managed to write *Dr. Jekyll and Mr. Hyde*, *Kidnapped*, and *A Child's Garden of Verses*. In August 1887, he set off on yet another health-seeking voyage; he settled at the famous Adirondack Cottage Sanitarium run by Edward Livingston Trudeau in Saranac, New York, for the winter of 1887–1888. Stevenson did not enjoy the local activities or other residents at the sanitarium, and he spent many hours in solitude, writing and smoking cigarettes. By April, Stevenson was well enough to travel again and his destination this time was the South Pacific. He and Fanny took up residence on a plantation in Samoa, where he enjoyed a short period of relatively good health. In 1893, he described his life with TB in a letter written to a friend; "For fourteen years I have not had a day's real health; I have awakened sick and gone to bed weary . . . I have written in bed, and written out of it, written in hemorrhages, written in sickness, written torn by coughing, written when my head swam for weakness." Ironically, the illness that had so greatly influenced his course in life would not be the one to strike the fatal blow. Stevenson died suddenly in 1894, at the age of 44, from what appears to have been a massive stroke, a cause that was apparently unrelated to his long battle with TB.

The way TB affected the literary giants Robert Louis Stevenson and John Keats is a contradiction in terms, illustrating two very different courses of the same illness. Keats recognized a sudden symptom of TB when he saw blood on his pillow, and within less than one year's time the disease had claimed his life. After his illness began, his literary productivity suffered and his rapid decline in health marked the end of his career even before it marked the end of his life. Stevenson, on the other hand, suffered through a life of chronic illness and relapsing symptoms, always on the move to find a cure. During his times of well-being he wrote prolifically, becoming a successful and admired author. In spite of the fact that TB influenced Stevenson's entire life, it was a sudden event with traumatic consequences, rather than TB, that brought about his untimely end. TB has an unpredictable nature that is influenced by many factors and in the case of these

---

Requiem by Robert Louis Stevenson (1879)

Fifteen years before died, during one of his periods of tuberculous illness when he was distraught and close to death, Stevenson wrote this poem, which is engraved on his tombstone. He is buried on a hillside in Samoa.

> Under the wide and starry sky
> Dig the grave and let me lie:
> Glad did I live and gladly die,
> And I laid me down with a will.
> This be the verse you grave for me:
> Here he lies where he longed to be:
> Home is the sailor, home from sea,
> And the hunter home from the hill.

two writers, the same disease led them each on a different path to early death—Keats's route was short and direct, while Stevenson took a long journey filled with many voyages and stops along the way.

While characters and plotlines frequently reflected the experience of TB when the author was personally afflicted with the disease, TB as a more general theme is found in the other fictional works as well. Many authors recognized the social and humanistic importance of TB and used it metaphorically in their work to represent the concept of suffering, inequality, and injustice. Patients who suffered from TB were frequently characters in the literature of Fyodor Dostoevsky, the 19th-century Russian writer. French author Victor Hugo represented the subject of TB in his 1862 novel of social injustice and despair, *Les Misérables*. One of the most influential works of 20th-century German literature, *The Magic Mountain*, by Thomas Mann (1924) takes place in a sanatorium high up in the Swiss Alps where all the characters suffer from TB. The sanatorium that is used as the setting of *The Magic Mountain* is the same place where Robert Louis Stevenson spent two years recuperating from an episode of TB. As late as 1990, Kurt Vonnegut used TB as a literary device to illustrate the themes of powerlessness and personal imprisonment in his novel *Hocus Pocus*.

A more contemporary turn on the age-old subject of TB is taken in John le Carré's 2001 novel *The Constant Gardener*, a story about an anti-TB drug that is being tested on unsuspecting people in the poverty-stricken slums of Nairobi, Kenya. This fictional account of murder and political corruption is set against the backdrop of TB control in a developing nation. In spite of the fact that the novel is a work of fiction, le Carré pushed real social and political hot buttons with his story; the book was originally banned in Kenya, a country in crisis with epidemic levels of TB. The novel and its namesake 2006 Academy Award–winning movie tell the story of a widower who is determined to unravel the mystery of his wife's murder and how it relates to government corruption and a powerful pharmaceutical company.

TUBERCULOSIS ON THE STAGE

The representation of TB across the eras is also reflected in art forms other than literature. The historical significance of TB is reflected in the plotlines of two of the most popular operas of all time, *La Bohème* by Giacomo Puccini (1896) and *La Traviata* by Giuseppe Verdi (1853). The respective heroine of each opera, Mimi in *La Bohème* and Violetta in *La Traviata*, sings a dramatic deathbed aria as consumption claims her young life and brings down the curtain on the show. Today, *La Bohème* is the second most frequently performed opera in the United States, even though TB is no longer a focal point of life for most Americans.

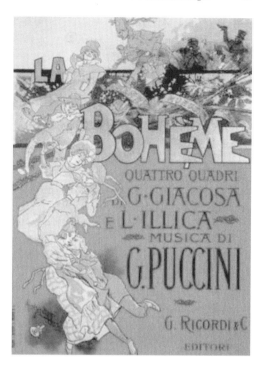

Poster for the 1896 production of Giacomo Puccini's *La Bohème.* Mimi, the heroine of the opera, sings a deathbed aria as TB brings the curtain down on her life and on the show.

Dying of TB Opera-Style

Dying of TB for the theatrical purpose of opera is an ironic portrayal of a disease that steals the breath away. In *La Traviata,* the soprano heroine Violetta is enfeebled and dying of TB. She coughs between musical notes and withers away with disease during the final scenes of her performance. For dramatic emphasis as the moment of death approaches, Violetta utters the only nonsung words in the opera, declaring that the pain is gone and she is once again free. As she is slipping away, the victim of a disease that destroys the lungs and causes incapacitating weakness, Violetta bolts upright in bed and manages to belt out the final aria of the opera before she dies and the curtain falls. When it comes to death from pulmonary TB, drama and reality could not be more different.

TB has transcended historical periods and has been artistically recreated on the stage for modern audiences. The Jonathan Larson Broadway stage production and 2005 film *Rent* were inspired by the story told in *La Bohème,* even though a contemporary twist was added to make the story more relevant to its time. To place the plot in a current frame of reference for American audiences, Larson uses the modern-day plague AIDS instead of TB as the disease of destiny for his cast of characters. Ironically, as AIDS assumed the lead role in *Rent* because of its contemporary impact, TB and AIDS became real costars in the world of infectious disease. TB and AIDS co-infection creates illness and destruction that are beyond what either disease can cause alone. The Pulitzer Prize–winning rock musical opened on Broadway in 1996, presenting the compelling story of a group of poor, young artists and musicians in New York whose creative struggles and fight for survival take place in a world overshadowed by the presence of AIDS.

TB takes another turn on stage in the musical *Les Misérables*, based on the Victor Hugo novel published in 1862. Musically staged for the first time in 1980 in Paris, *Les Misérables* is an all-encompassing story of social injustice, love, the law, good, evil, and morality. Once again, TB causes the death of a main character and becomes a defining moment in the plot of the story, reflective of the character of the disease in the lives of those who suffered and the societies in which it occurred.

In the genre of nonmusical theater, *Long Day's Journey Into Night*, written by American playwright Eugene O'Neill, is an autobiographical drama that portrays one day in the life of a dysfunctional family that is plagued by alcoholism and drug addiction. In the midst of conflict, additional stress is introduced when the son is diagnosed with TB. Written in 1940, O'Neill instructed that it not be published until after his death. It ultimately made its debut in 1956, three years after O'Neill died. Widely considered to be his finest work, he posthumously received the 1957 Pulitzer Prize for Drama for his play.

TUBERCULOSIS IN THE MOVIES

Similar to the way the story of *La Bohème* was updated and retold in *Rent*, the timeless plot of *La Traviata* was recreated in 2001 to become the basis of the pop culture hit and Oscar-winning musical-drama *Moulin Rouge!* starring Nicole Kidman and Ewan McGregor. Populated with music from a variety of familiar 20th-century sources, the movie is set in 1899 and tells the story of a young British poet who moves to Paris and becomes involved in a dangerous love triangle. The beautiful nightclub star who becomes the object of his passion is unaware that she is dying of TB, a force even greater than love.

Long Day's Journey Into Night was made into a critically acclaimed movie in 1962; Katharine Hepburn, who starred as the morphine-addicted wife and mother of the family, was nominated for the Academy Award for Best Actress for her performance. Other relatively recent films have also used the theme of TB as a dramatic device to tell their stories. *Midnight Cowboy,* with Dustin Hoffman and Jon Voight (1969); *Heavenly Creatures,* with Kate Winslet (1994); *Tombstone,* with Val Kilmer and Kurt Russell (1993); *The End of the Affair,* with Ralph Fiennes and Julianne Moore (1999); and *There Will Be Blood,* with Daniel Day Lewis are some of the more contemporary movies that have a plot point or character that is associated with TB.

TUBERCULOSIS SINGS THE BLUES

TB has been represented in various forms of music throughout history, both thematically, as in opera, and by the many composers who were afflicted with the disease. In America, TB in music is perhaps best represented in the style known as the blues. The blues emerged from the spirituals, work songs, and ballads sung in African American communities throughout the country. Blues singers often expressed their concerns and worries through their music, so it is no wonder that songs about TB emerged from the blues tradition. As TB spread rampantly throughout America in the 1920s, no single group was more affected than African Americans. When the words "everybody spit in your face ain't friend to you" were sung by blues singer Jim Jackson, the double-edged message clearly referred to the heartbreak of TB among African Americans and the effect it had on its victims and their families.

"TB Blues," written and recorded by blues singer and songwriter Victoria Spivey (1906–1976) in 1927, was one of many songs that grew out of the African American experience of suffering and apprehension in relation to the devastating disease. In the distinctive style of the blues, the song immortalized what it felt like to have TB. As the disease continued to overwhelm African Americans, Spivey continued to sing about it, telling more of the story in subsequent songs like "Dirty TB Blues" and "TB's Got Me." The relationship between TB and the blues emerged again in 1963 when the famous jazz pianist Bud Powell was treated for TB at the Bouffemont sanatorium in France, where he wrote the well-known song "Blues for Bouffemont."

Jimmie Rodgers (1897–1933) is described by many as "the Father of Country Music" and the first star of rock and roll. In his song also entitled "TB Blues" as well as in "My Time Ain't Long," he chronicled his experience with TB. He foreshadowed his imminent death from TB through his song lyrics: "I've got that old TB I can't eat a bite, got me worried so I can't even sleep at night, I've got the TB blues." After a short six-year career during which he sang about his disease, he died from TB in 1933. More recent songs, such as Van Morrison's "TB Sheets" (1974), have also captured the experience of TB and kept the theme of TB alive in American music.

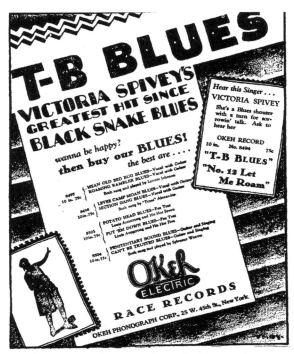

An advertisement for "TB Blues," by Victoria Spivey,
from the *Chicago Defender* newspaper on November 19,
1927. In the tradition of the blues, Spivey sang about TB
in many of her songs. Courtesy of the *Chicago Defender*.

TUBERCULOSIS ON CANVAS

TB made an artistic impression in the world of painting and helped to define
the portrayal of changing social class values. Artists from 19th-century Europe
could not escape the ravages of TB any better than the rest of society, so it is not a
surprise that it became the subject of their obsessions, their inspirations, and their
work. While experiences with illness and death are very personal, the attitudes
and behaviors associated with them are also the product of the era during which
they occur and the social class of the victim. The ruling classes of 19th-century
Europe tended to experience illness, including TB, more through the lens of family, clan, and lineage than from an individual perspective.

An example of death and ruling class values in the 19th century can be found
in the story of Joséphine Eléonore Marie Pauline de Galard de Brassacede Béarn,

the Princesse de Broglie. A member of the most cultivated circles of the French Second Empire, the princess was renowned for her great beauty and she is remembered as being the last society woman who commissioned a portrait from the renowned painter Jean-Auguste-Dominique Ingres (1780–1867). Shortly after the portrait was completed, Princesse de Broglie died of consumption at the age of 35 and it is said that her bereaved husband kept the painting behind draperies in perpetual tribute to her memory. While the death of Princesse de Broglie was surely mourned by her family, her loss was also most likely tempered by the mindset of a social class that considered her earthly duty fulfilled when she gave birth to an heir to the family's dukedom. The Ingres painting remained in the family until it was sold in 1975.

As newly forming middle-class values changed the prevailing ruling-class attitudes in Europe, the concept of honoring an individual's illness and death emerged with society's new structure. Death from TB became personal tragedy in the new middle class. When the prodigious painter Edvard Munch (1863–1944) lost his young sister Sophie to TB in 1877, his life and his work were forever changed. Born into the emerging European middle class, Munch's experiences with TB became a focal point of his painting and a reflection of his upbringing. The very personal portrayals of Munch's relationship with TB mark the beginning of a middle-class value regarding illness and death.

When Munch was a child, he was often ill and kept out of school during the long, cold winters in Oslo. In his solitude, Munch would draw to keep himself occupied. Munch's father was a doctor. He was a loving but extremely nervous and obsessively religious man. The oppressive atmosphere of the home, Munch's poor health, and a nighttime ritual of reading vivid ghost stories stimulated Munch's active imagination and brought on bizarre visions and nightmares. He felt the constant presence of death. To add to the specter of illness in the household, another younger sister was diagnosed with mental illness at an early age, leading Munch to later write: "I inherited two of mankind's most frightful enemies—the heritage of consumption and insanity." Perhaps his most famous painting, *The Scream* (1893) illustrates the effect both of these illnesses had on Munch.

His 1885 painting *The Sick Child* most clearly reflects his experiences with TB. Completed early in his career when he was only 22 years old, Munch painted the image several times in an attempt to capture what he remembered seeing when young Sophie died—"the pale transparent skin against the linen sheets, the trembling lips, the shaking hands." The theme of a sick child became one of Munch's most powerful subjects, which he explored in various media between 1885 and 1896. Munch's personal memories, including the death of his mother, the trauma of his sister's death, and visits to dying patients with his father, are clearly reflected in his works. He described *The Sick Child* as "a breakthrough in my art." He painted several subsequent versions of the original painting and also expressed the haunting image of TB in *Spring*, painted a few years later. Irreplaceable personal loss at the hands of TB became the foundation of a tragically inspired career and a poignantly difficult life.

Andrew Wyeth (1917–2009) was one of the best-known American artists of the middle 20th century. Most commonly referred to as a visual artist, he painted in a realist style, frequently using his surroundings as the subject of his work. Wyeth's favorite subject for landscape painting was his immediate environment, either the area around his home in Chadds Ford, Pennsylvania, or the town where he spent his summers, Cushing, Maine. Wyeth was sometimes called the "Painter of the People" because his work was so popular with the American public. One of the most well-known images in 20th-century American art is his painting *Christina's World*, which is currently housed in the collection of the Museum of Modern Art in New York City.

Because Wyeth was a very thin and nervous child, his parents took him out of school after the third grade and arranged for him to be tutored at home. Although the cause of his frailty was originally diagnosed as a sinus illness, it was later discovered that the condition that kept him away from his school and friends was TB. In his solitude, he wandered and played in the hills around his home, painting in watercolor and drawing. His childhood art exploded with unrestrained exuberance that he later described as "slapdash" and "wild and undisciplined." As he grew older, his artistic talent was reigned in and refined by his father, who was a painter and illustrator. To Wyeth's father, there was value in finding interest in even the most mundane objects of everyday life and he advocated that his son pay attention to the subtle influences of the natural world by living around it, in it, and as part of it.

As Wyeth grew older, his painting acquired a more intense emotional tone, and he began to paint figures, mostly portraits of single people. *Trodden Weed*

Edvard Munch on *The Sick Child*

"The only influences in *The Sick Child* were the ones that came from my home…my childhood and my home. Only someone who knew the conditions at home could possibly understand why there can be no conceivable chance of any other place having played a part—my home is to my art as a midwife is to her children…few painters have ever experienced the full grief of their subject as I did in *The Sick Child*. It was not just I who was suffering, it was all my nearest and dearest as well." (Prideaux, 2007)

(1951), a painting that is said to have been admired by Nikita Khrushchev, a leader in the Soviet Union from 1953 to 1964, portrays only a man's booted legs walking across the grass. This work was intended to be a self-portrait; it was conceived while Wyeth was recuperating from surgery to remove part of a lung that was damaged by his early bout with TB.

Wyeth brought intense personal associations, meaning, and emotion to the people and objects he painted. His early experiences with illness and solitude greatly influenced the paintings he produced. During one of his trips to Maine, Wyeth met Christina Olson, a severely disabled neighbor who had an undiagnosed muscular weakening that paralyzed her lower body. Wyeth was greatly intrigued and inspired by her strength and perseverance, and during their long friendship he used her as a model in several paintings.

Christina's World (1948) is perhaps the most famous of all Wyeth's paintings. He was inspired to create it when he saw Christina crawling up a sloping hillside toward her home. The image of the crippled girl, alone and struggling, became his inspired subject matter. He painted her body so that her face is turned away from view. Wyeth vividly renders Christina's twisted body, rigid arm, disabled legs, and dark, wind-blown hair. In Christina, Wyeth captures the experience of living life from the point of view of the wounded and the lonely. Perhaps this vision was cultivated in his own early experience with TB. In *Christina's World,* he painted "the loneliness of that figure—perhaps the same that I felt myself as a kid."

Wyeth painted Christina on numerous occasions, portraying the nature of illness and disability and the isolation that is often associated with it. In his empathic portraits of his friend's physical disability, the painter characterizes the limits that are imposed by physical illness, the difficulty of imagining what lies beyond the limits, and the beauty and light that can be achieved by living in relation to them. The limitations that defined life for Christina were undiagnosed and misunderstood. For Wyeth, the illness that created boundaries, isolation, and insight for him had a name—it was TB.

RAISING AWARENESS THROUGH THE ARTS

TB in the arts has become important beyond its thematic contributions, its social commentaries, and its effect on artists through the ages. The arts have now become an avenue for increasing awareness of the global impact of TB and a contributor to the goal of worldwide eradication of the disease through a program called the Stop TB Partnership. Established in 2000, the Partnership operates with the immediate objective of eliminating TB as a public health problem and an ultimate goal of creating a world that is free of TB. It is the hope of the Partnership that the first children born in this millennium will see TB eradicated in their lifetime. The Partnership relies on a network of more than 700 international organizations, countries, public and private donors, patient organizations, and nongovernmental and governmental organizations to work together to achieve these goals. Several Partnership programs have used the arts as a means of drawing attention to the problem of TB.

The longstanding link between TB and music has been used to raise global awareness of TB through a Stop TB Partnership project called Music to Stop TB. In 2008, for example, Stop TB partners in Canada performed a series of TB outreach activities using a combination of musical entertainment and education. To raise awareness about TB among people who love opera and to inspire a love of opera among people who are committed to the global fight against TB, Opera Lyra Ottawa paired TB education with performances of *La Traviata*. Ambassadors representing countries facing a high TB burden, members of the Canadian Parliament, TB experts, community representatives, and local citizens interested in the arts gathered to enjoy the opera and to learn about why the global TB crisis is an issue Canadians should care about. Music to Stop TB also raises TB consciousness through concerts featuring compositions by Frédéric Chopin (who died of TB at age 39), Luigi Boccherini, Giovanni Battista Pergolesi, and other composers who died of TB. This novel advocacy approach was designed to raise TB awareness by mobilizing the universal love of music.

The Images to Stop TB Photo Award, also launched in 2008, was initiated to raise TB awareness through an international photography contest featuring images of TB prevention, treatment, and community activity. This award was organized in collaboration with institutions and organizations that specialize in photography, and the contest winner was chosen by an international jury of photography experts, representatives from the United Nations, and other partnering organizations. The winner received a grant to take a series of photos that are featured in a photo exhibition that tours the world to raise TB awareness. Each photograph in the exhibit was taken in one of the 22 countries that are most heavily affected by TB (Afghanistan, Bangladesh, Brazil, Cambodia, China, Democratic Republic of Congo, Ethiopia, India, Indonesia, Kenya, Mozambique, Myanmar, Nigeria, Pakistan, Philippines, Russian Federation, South Africa, Thailand, Uganda, United Republic of Tanzania, Vietnam, or Zimbabwe). Through the contest and the exhibition, an array of international photographers and emerging young talents embraced yet another art form to capture both the suffering and the hope of those affected by TB.

Just as celebrities and politicians put their public personas behind the Christmas Seal advocacy effort in decades gone by, an international soccer player from Portugal has made stopping TB one of his goals. Luís Figo, who is considered by many fans to be one of the greatest professional soccer players of all time, used his athletic fame and status to launch the "I Am Stopping Tuberculosis" campaign. Aimed at children and young adults who are his biggest fans, Figo's initiative raises awareness by distributing computer wallpapers, posters, and postcards that deliver key messages about TB. In conjunction with this campaign, the Stop TB Partnership is capitalizing on Figo's image by producing a 16-page educational comic book about TB featuring the soccer player as the main character. The comic book was drawn by an artist who was chosen by a jury of international cartoon experts and representatives from the United Nations in yet another artistic competition that began in 2008. The resulting comic book represents one more artistic genre that has been claimed by TB, this time focusing the spotlight of TB awareness on the young people of the world.

7

Resurgence of the Social Disease: Tuberculosis Makes a Comeback

TB is not merely an infectious disease. It is more than just a biological process that consists of bacteria, contagion, immune response, infection, and disease. As has been demonstrated throughout the ages, TB exists in a broader socioeconomic and political environment. It is a social disease—it has always existed locally in a context that is heavily influenced by ecological, economic, political, and cultural factors that manipulate the likelihood of developing the disease. Medicine cannot override the power of social forces and the impact of local environments; these factors have to be recognized so that intervention to stop TB can address diverse factors in global neighborhoods and become the foundation for progress.

THE SOCIAL DISEASE

Public health authorities and medical experts believed that the discovery of antibiotics that were effective against M. *tuberculosis* would be the beginning of the end for the disease that had held humans hostage since the beginning of human history. They were wrong. TB defied the expectations of the experts and to this day it remains a leading cause of global infectious illness and death, despite the existence of effective and inexpensive treatment. The development of TB strains that are resistant to anti-TB drugs, in addition to challenging social and economic conditions in developing and impoverished nations, have contributed to a worldwide resurgence of TB. Poverty, institutional living conditions, displacement of refugees due to war and political instability, HIV/AIDS, and immigration patterns are social factors that play a role in the continuing story of TB. Effective treatment for all people and attention to the sociopolitical environments that hinder TB control are needed to quell the epidemic that still rages in some parts of the world.

Significant differences in the outcomes of TB, including the likelihood of death from the disease, exist in close relation to race, ethnicity, and place of birth. These disparities are related to the social and economic conditions of the affected groups, not to any innate biological variation among people. The correlation between socioeconomic circumstances and TB has been recognized for a long time. Malnutrition, overcrowding, and limited access to medical care are all factors that are associated with poverty, as well as with an increased risk of becoming infected with TB and of developing active TB.

Between the mid-19th and the mid-20th centuries, there was a significant decline in the incidence of TB in developed countries. Because antibiotics that could treat TB were introduced around the time that TB was already declining, most of the credit for decreasing rates of disease was given to the newly available medical treatments. Although several social factors also contributed to the drop in TB incidence, they were largely unappreciated in light of the miracle of medicine. During this time, however, improved socioeconomic conditions, including better working conditions, less overcrowding, advancing public health measures, increased awareness of how germs spread, and education also contributed to reduced TB transmission and infection.

Poverty and TB go hand in glove. In one district of India, for example, people who earned less than the equivalent of $7 (US) per month had two times higher TB prevalence than those earning more than $20 (US) per month (World Health Organization, 2001). However, poverty is not a factor that exclusively influences TB prevalence in developing nations. In the developed world as well, people living in poverty are also more likely to live in conditions that are conducive to TB. For example, poverty in developed nations is associated with worse access to health care, which leads to delayed TB diagnosis. Among the poor, if TB is diagnosed and antibiotics are prescribed, there is a greater likelihood that treatment will be inconsistent or incomplete, leaving poor patients at risk for relapse and the development of multidrug-resistant strains of bacteria. TB frequently affects young adults during their most economically productive time of life; the loss of productivity due to illness and time lost from work makes the socioeconomic burden of TB a particularly serious problem.

Higher rates of TB among minorities and immigrants in developed countries are the result of several social conditions. In industrialized nations, racial and ethnic minorities are disproportionately affected by social and economic conditions, such as low income, lack of access to health care, prison confinement, and unemployment, that are conducive to higher rates of TB. In places such as the United States, Australia, and Western Europe, where there are higher TB rates among minorities and immigrants than among native-born people, a public health dilemma has been created. How can governments and public health agencies effectively deal with the different rates of TB among minorities while maintaining nondiscriminatory disease control policies and practices? The answer lies in the ability to improve the social factors that encourage TB to thrive. This is an essential component of international TB control.

PUBLIC HEALTH ATTITUDES IN THE EARLY POST-ANTIBIOTIC YEARS

By the 1950s, public health officials in the United States viewed infectious diseases, TB among them, as problems of the past. Medical students were actively encouraged to focus their studies on areas of medicine that would be more relevant in the future than infectious disease. TB rates began to decline in the United States and after several years of steady improvement, the Department of Health and Human Services predicted that TB would be eliminated in the United States by 2010. The development of anti-TB drugs had created complacency among public health agencies and TB control programs, which contributed to the belief that infectious disease would no longer be an important cause of sickness and death in the near future.

Early optimism regarding the fate of infectious disease was short-lived, however, and health officials were forced to re-examine their position when new epidemics of old diseases such as cholera and malaria struck parts of the world in the 1960s and 1970s. In addition, more than 30 new infectious diseases, including Lyme disease, Ebola virus, HIV/AIDS, and the H1N1 swine flu, have emerged in human populations since 1973. Infectious diseases, both new and old, with the potential for worldwide disease pandemics, remain a significant health concern everywhere.

Through many decades of the 20th century, most industrialized nations enjoyed a decline in the rate of TB occurrence because of the availability of effective treatment and improved social conditions. Many middle-income nations, such as Algeria, Chile, and Cuba, were able to follow the trend of decreasing TB by introducing widespread disease control strategies that managed infection with antibiotic treatment and enhanced patient support. The good times would be short-lived, however, and as the 1980s dawned, the world faced yet another resurgence of TB and the end of the steadily declining global rates that had been enjoyed in response to antibiotic treatment. The reversal of TB decline can be blamed on several factors; diminished public health efforts, shifting patterns of global poverty, the increasing emergence of drug-resistant strains, and the spread of HIV all contributed to the devastating global turn-around and increasing incidence of TB. Developing nations around the world have been especially affected by the wild spread and dramatic increase in the rate of TB because of population growth, failing economies, and ineffective national TB control programs. However, the stories of TB resurgence in the developed nations of the world also have plotlines that illustrate the intricate relationship between TB and society regardless of where it occurs.

THE RESURGENCE OF TUBERCULOSIS IN THE UNITED STATES

Even though the brunt of the TB resurgence in recent years has been experienced in developing nations of the world, industrialized countries have not been immune to the comeback. After 30 years of stable decline in the United States, TB once again earned public attention with a 20 percent increase in the rate of disease between 1985 and 1992 (Centers for Disease Control, 2006–2007).

TB came back to New York City when it was least expected. Its resurgence and transmission serve as a good example of how an epidemic develops. In 1968, after so many years of decline, city and health authorities envisioned a TB-free New York. They recommended closing hospital beds that had been reserved for TB patients and planned to rely on anti-TB drugs for control of the few errant cases that occurred each year. The first sign of trouble came in 1975 and 1976, when the number of new cases of TB unexpectedly rose for two years in a row. This increase may have initially been dismissed as a statistical fluke, especially since it was followed by extremely rapid decline in new cases over the next two years.

In 1978, New York City recorded the lowest number of new TB cases in its history (Gandy, 2003). However, hope that the two years of increased TB had just been a fluke faded when, in 1979, the rate of new TB cases began a consistent upward trend that signaled the start of an epidemic. The incidence of TB rose throughout the 1980s in New York City, but little was done to address the problem. By 1990, city officials had been aware of epidemic rates of new TB cases for several years but their delayed acknowledgement of the problem added to the already enormous burden of TB in the city. In little more than a decade, how did TB go from near-extinction to epidemic proportions in New York City?

New York City is divided into 30 health districts. In 1978, the year of historically low citywide TB, traditionally poor districts with large African American

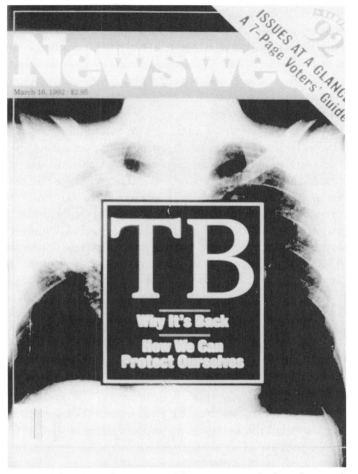

Cover of *Newsweek* from March 16, 1992. The resurgence of tuberculosis in the United States in the 1980s was viewed as an emerging threat to the health of the nation. Courtesy of the Centers for Disease Control and Prevention.

populations had the heaviest concentrations of TB cases, and other poor, racially distinct districts began to record an elevation in new TB cases. In 1979, the incidence of new cases became highly concentrated in large neighborhoods in the most affected districts, suggesting that, just as a hurricane gathers strength and forms an eye, the epidemic was forming its center. Soon disease began to spread to other districts that were susceptible because they contained a high density of TB-vulnerable people. As a continued process of infection and contagion was established between the central area of disease and TB-susceptible neighborhoods, a second, and then a third, area of intense TB concentration developed. When the already vulnerable poor and minority neighborhoods were fully saturated with TB, the disease began to seep across the imaginary health district boundaries to affect other populations. It wasn't long before epidemic levels of new TB cases could be found in all but the wealthiest areas of New York City as TB spread throughout the community.

In order for an epidemic to continue, disease transmission must occur both at the community level and within households. New TB cases among preschool children served as the indicator of transmission among family members since young children are less likely to have extensive social contact outside the family. Early in the epidemic, the rate of new cases of TB among preschoolers was strongly correlated with the rate of new cases among African American and Hispanic adults, suggesting that the spread of TB was occurring within households in these groups. By 1990, white children under the age of five began to experience higher levels of TB than had been recorded in earlier years, indicating that the epidemic had crossed racial boundaries. Community and household transmission was taking place in a large number of New York City health districts, supporting the spread of TB infection, its progression to active disease, and the continuation of the epidemic.

Because TB resources had been drastically minimized during the years of TB decline, New York City was dreadfully unprepared to deal with the epidemic number of new cases. In order to defeat the epidemic, the city almost exclusively relied on the use of anti-TB drugs. A well-funded DOTS program, the short-course directly observed therapy plan, was initiated in 1993 and large numbers of people received anti-TB drugs. New TB cases began to decline and most health authorities attributed the improvement to the success of the DOTS program. In reality, TB incidence had already peaked and begun to slow by 1993, and although extensive use of antibiotics no doubt played a large role in suppressing the TB epidemic, additional dynamics helped to restrain TB. No successful TB control effort can rely on antibiotics alone; expanded case finding, legislation to ensure treatment compliance, increased public funding, and public health efforts were also used to help control the resurgence of TB.

Between 1975 and 1993, tens of thousands of New Yorkers from all ethnicities, classes, ages, and levels of education were affected by a modern-day epidemic of an ancient disease. Then, in a turn of events that mimics the rise and fall of TB through the centuries, the number of new TB cases in New York City began to fall. The unexpected TB surge in New York caused a city to pause and re-evaluate the factors that contributed to it and the measures that were necessary to control a controllable disease. Even though TB eventually crossed socioeconomic barriers to affect all but the wealthiest areas of the city, increasing poverty among the urban poor, the impact of HIV, drug abuse, homelessness, inadequate public health support to control TB, and increasing immigration from countries where TB was highly prevalent were the factors that allowed TB to regain its foothold in New York. In spite of the relative wealth enjoyed by the United States, socioeconomic conditions such as these are not uncommon in many urban areas. These factors are not unlike the circumstances that exist in impoverished and politically unstable nations around the world where TB continues to thrive in spite of the availability of a cure.

The epidemic in New York City indicated to public health officials across the United States that the infrastructure of TB control had broken down during the years of complacence about TB and other infectious diseases. In response, resources at national, state, and local levels were increased to help stop the resurgence of TB. Early identification of TB cases, treatment of latent TB in cases that had a high risk of becoming active disease, and the use of case management strategies, including more widespread use of DOTS, to increase the rate of therapy completion were employed to address increasing TB prevalence in the United States. The effort paid off—between 1993 and 2003, a 44 percent decline in TB incidence was documented in the United States (Gandy, 2003).

Currently, the United States enjoys historically low rates of TB. In spite of this, however, overall progress toward eliminating TB in the United States has slowed in recent years. One of the reasons for the slowing rate of decline is the number of TB cases among foreign-born people who live in the United States. In 2007, the TB rate was 9.7 percent higher for foreign-born people living in the United States than for people born in the United States (Centers for Disease Control, Trends in Tuberculosis, 2008). In an effort to address the higher rate of TB among people who were not born in the United States, new medical screening requirements have been adopted for people requesting to immigrate from foreign countries with high rates of TB. Beyond immigration-related issues, racial and ethnic minorities in general carry more than their share of the burden of TB in the United States. The incidence of TB is several times higher among Hispanic, black, and Asian individuals than among whites. In 2007, the greatest difference in TB rates among racial groups born in the United States was between African Americans and whites, with the TB rate nearly eight times higher among African Americans.

THE RESURGENCE OF TUBERCULOSIS IN THE UNITED KINGDOM

TB also made a comeback late in the 20th century in London, the scene of such utter TB destruction and despair in the 19th century. The story of TB in modern London is a story of how disease intersects with urban social conditions like poverty, homelessness, and immigration. Beginning in the late 1980s, TB case reports increased substantially and it is estimated that more than 50 people per week developed TB in London. Of all the cases of TB reported in England and Wales, 40 percent of all cases and 50 percent of drug-resistant cases were found in the city of London (Gandy, 2003). Increasing disparity between the wealthy and the poor, homelessness, HIV/TB co-infection, migration, and neglect of TB prevention and control services were factors that contributed to making the population of London vulnerable to TB once again. Except for during the two world wars, Londoners had enjoyed rapidly declining levels of TB since the early 1900s. Improved housing conditions, better nutrition, and better health care in general helped to support decreasing levels of TB until 1988, when the rate of decline began to even out. Effective antibiotic treatment for TB meant that patients could be treated and cured at home, so sanatoria throughout Britain closed and TB specialist services faded away. But when the environmental and social circumstances were right, TB came roaring back.

In London, as in many big cities, there are great differences in the circumstances of the rich and the poor. As the economic gap between rich and poor in the United Kingdom grew wider, inequalities in the health of the population followed suit. Poverty has been highlighted as one of the major reasons for the increasing number of TB cases in London. Since 1988, increasing rates of TB have been reported in the poorest 30 percent of the people in England and Wales, but not in the remainder of the population. Additionally, overcrowding increased by 40 percent in London between 1984 and 1997, giving TB more opportunity to flourish since poverty and substandard housing conditions, or homelessness, are among the circumstances that allow TB to thrive.

War, environmental disasters, and human rights violations in various parts of the world have caused many people to flee their homelands in the last quarter of the 20th century. Immigration to London from countries with high endemic TB rates has undoubtedly been a factor in the rise of TB in the city. To combat the effects immigration has on rising levels of TB, the government enforces strict TB screening for people entering Britain from countries where the disease is common. Although this type of active screening helps to identify people with TB before they enter the general population of London, effective TB control also requires access to health care services in the communities where refugees may settle. Refugee communities tend to receive poor health care in London and, as a result, refugees tend to suffer from poor physical and mental health. Delayed treatment seeking after the onset of TB symptoms, increased transmission of the disease, more serious health consequences, and poor use of preventive measures such as the treatment of latent TB are problems that arise in the absence of good overall health care for immigrants.

London has one of the highest rates of homelessness in Europe. Dealing with TB among homeless people is associated with several difficult challenges. Unlike the United States, health care in the United Kingdom is nationalized and administered by the National Health Service. In the mid-1990s, between 25 percent and 37 percent of homeless people in the United Kingdom were not registered to receive health care, meaning that homeless people not only have worse health than the general public but they also have less access to health care (Gandy, 2003). Homeless people with TB who manage to navigate the bureaucracy and gain access to health care usually present with more advanced and more infectious forms of disease. Because of the length and complexity of TB treatment, it is not surprising that significant numbers of homeless people who are diagnosed with TB fail to complete treatment.

In the United Kingdom, DOTS is recommended for all patients who are likely to have difficulty taking the prescribed TB treatment regimen. Programs that encourage treatment adherence and offer support to homeless people with TB are very important—studies show that 80 percent of homeless people with TB in London can achieve a cure with the help of skilled outreach workers, incentive programs such as food or transportation vouchers, and a collaborative approach to treatment (Gandy, 2003). Like other large metropolitan areas around the world, London is looking for ways to improve TB prevention, treatment, and control. Regardless of where TB appears, social circumstances produce the fertile environment in which TB grows and the effort to combat the disease must include attention to the socioeconomic circumstances that allow it to thrive.

TUBERCULOSIS IN PRISONS: THE STATES OF THE FORMER SOVIET UNION

As in many other places in the world, the history of Russia and the Soviet Union can be told in parallel with a history of TB. In czarist Russia, TB was a massive problem made even worse by the fact that no coherent public health system existed to attempt to control it. Before World War I, death from TB in Russia occurred at a rate of 400 per 100,000 people. During the war, 1.7 million Russian soldiers were killed in fighting, but more than 2 million civilians died of TB (Gandy, 2003). Even though increased rates of TB were seen immediately after the war in the wake of social upheaval, the formation of a centralized, nationwide network to control TB became entwined with the birth of the Soviet Union.

Organized TB care was a priority of the fledgling postwar Soviet Union and resources to control it were used to create sanatoria, mass screening programs, and BCG vaccination programs. Additionally, the government maintained a modest standard of living for its citizens by providing ready employment, education, and basic food supplies thereby creating a less than ideal environment in which TB could thrive. By the 1970s, TB in the Soviet Union was rare. In 1989, just before the end of the communist era, the rate of TB was 44.7 cases per 100,000 people (Gandy, 2003). The end of the Soviet Union was both the end of a way of life for the people who lived there and the beginning of yet another TB epidemic. Some of the reasons why a new TB epidemic emerged at this time are clear and reminiscent of the reasons that TB occurs anywhere. The end of communism and the transition to a market economy meant that millions of people were suddenly plunged into poverty as formerly stable employment was lost. Civil wars erupted, the health care sector was dismantled, and crime increased, as did the demand for punishment of the criminals. Of all the social factors that contributed to new epidemic levels of TB in the former Soviet states, institutional living within the prison system was the key. The story of the TB in Russia is ultimately a story of TB behind bars.

Post-Soviet social change was accompanied by increased poverty, which caused increased crime and fear, and an increased public demand for better protection. As a result, arrest rates in former Soviet states tripled between 1988 and 1995, and the prison population exploded. By 2000, the Russian Federation and some other former Soviet states had imprisonment rates that were among the highest in the world. In spite of reforms and the adoption of international human rights standards in the criminal justice systems of Eastern Europe, the impact of massive prison overcrowding created appalling conditions. In the mid-1990s, the International Committee of the Red Cross visited prisoners in Baku, Azerbaijan, and revealed that dangerous levels of TB infection were occurring. The Red Cross and Médecins Sans Frontières (Doctors without Borders), another international heath care organization, began TB control programs. In 1998, 1 in 10 Russian prisoners was suffering from active TB and an estimated 20,000 had multidrug-resistant cases (Gandy, 2003).

Prison conditions are ideal for the spread of TB—generally speaking, TB is 100 times more common in prison than in civilian populations. Many people enter prison already infected with TB and it is easily transmitted in a prison environment. In 1999, it was estimated that one-third of all the TB cases in Russia were found in prisons and in some cases, the vagaries of Russian prison life added to the already immense burden of TB. For example, there are small windows in the cells of prisons throughout the former Soviet Union that are, by law, covered on the outside with heavy metal shutters. The shutters are there to prevent contact between prisoners—if prisoners cannot shout to each other through the barrier of shutters, they cannot conspire with each other. The shutters, however, also prevent fresh air and light from penetrating into the cell from outside. When combined with the horrendous overcrowding that is endemic in Russian prisons, the closed shutters result in almost total lack of ventilation and extremely poor air quality, creating an ideal environment for the spread of TB. Despite epidemic levels of TB, however, the shutters in most Russian prisons remain closed and TB continues to thrive.

The spread of multidrug-resistant TB in Russian prisons has been a major cause of concern in large part because of the danger it poses to the civilian population at large. Estimates of the incidence of multidrug-resistant TB in Russian prisons differ but they are always high, ranging from 20 percent to a staggering 92 percent in one prison in Baku (Gandy, 2003). Since the former Soviet Union was not a developing nation and anti-TB drugs were available, why did multidrug-resistant TB become such an enormous problem in the prisons? Once again, several factors contributed to the problem. In prison, everything of value is traded and bartered—even medications that can save a prisoner's life are on the trading block. Anti-TB drugs were a valuable commodity in Soviet prisons and a flourishing black market in medications affected the consistent availability of treatment for those who needed it. This and other factors related to the reliability of the drug supply created an environment where many prisoners who had TB did not complete an adequate course of treatment, an important piece of the multidrug-resistant TB puzzle. Additionally, laboratory facilities were not available to test for drug resistance, so the correct antibiotics may not have been used for treatment in the first place. Even prisoners with known cases of multidrug-resistant TB were not isolated and as a result, others became infected with resistant strains of disease. The spread of HIV within the Russian prison population was also a contributing factor in the spread of TB, in general, and of multidrug-resistant strains, in particular.

The TB epidemic in Russian prisons raises many questions about human rights, social justice, and public health. Prison reform is an essential part of containing the TB epidemic within Russian prisons, a task much more easily discussed than accomplished. Issues related to health care, overcrowding, malnutrition, inequality, corruption, and injustice are enmeshed in prison life and in the TB epidemic.

Factors That Contribute to the Spread of TB in Prison

According to the World Health Organization, these are the factors that encourage the transmission of TB in prison: late case detection, lack of isolation to prevent contagion, inadequate treatment of people who are infectious, high prisoner turnover, overcrowding, poor ventilation, poor nutrition from prison food, and the physical and psychological stress of imprisonment.

Some changes have been made to attempt to contain the epidemic within the walls of the prisons, but the rate of infection is immense and the level of multi-drug-resistant cases demands more than DOTS can offer. In Azerbaijan, however, the law requiring that the small cell windows be covered with heavy shutters has been repealed, so at least a little light is shining in.

THE GLOBAL TUBERCULOSIS CRISIS

In 1993, the World Health Organization declared a "global health emergency" in response to the burgeoning occurrence of TB in developing countries. To cope with the crisis, greater support from governments in countries with epidemic TB rates and better international effort from the global community were called for. Currently, the TB epidemic continues to worsen in many places throughout the world and particularly urgent action is needed in several areas, most notably in Africa, Asia, and Eastern Europe.

In many areas where the TB epidemic rages on, human resources in the health care sector are already greatly overburdened. Health care in sub-Saharan Africa, for example, is immeasurably challenged by the rapid rise of TB cases that have been produced in association with epidemic levels of HIV. In Eastern Europe, the socioeconomic crisis that followed the dismantling of the Soviet Union in the early 1990s and impoverished public health systems have contributed to a major increase in the incidence and prevalence of TB, including cases of multidrug-resistant disease. Increased and sustained efforts toward TB control are also needed in Asia, which continues to bear two-thirds of the global burden of TB. Recent worldwide progress in TB control is threatened by an emerging HIV epidemic in Asia and outbreaks of multidrug-resistant disease in some parts of China.

In spite of the fact that M. *tuberculosis* was identified as the cause of TB more than a century ago and effective treatment has been available for more than half a century, a global public health crisis has developed and taken root. Because the world is a global community connected by international travel, business, and immigration, TB anywhere means TB everywhere. To control and eradicate TB globally, managing the social and political factors that encourage it to occur in developing nations becomes ever more important.

Tuberculosis and HIV Co-Infection

HIV and TB are the first and second most deadly infectious diseases in the world, respectively. In 2007, 2 million people died of HIV/AIDS and almost 1.8 million died of TB (Center for Global Health Policy, 2009). HIV/AIDS is a disease that suppresses immune function and attacks the very cells that are responsible for protecting people against TB. Impaired immune response greatly increases the risk that latent TB will be reactivated, in addition to making HIV-infected people more susceptible to new TB infection and rapid development of TB disease. HIV infection is associated with TB in children as well as in adults. In 2007, more than 30 million people worldwide were living with HIV infection, and approximately 2 billion people, or one-third of the world's population, were infected with M. *tuberculosis*.

The burden of HIV/TB co-infection is high; it is estimated that a third of the people living with HIV infection also have TB, and TB is the cause of death for as many as half of all people with AIDS. Since 1990, TB infection rates have increased fourfold in countries that are heavily affected by HIV (Centers for Disease Control, TB and HIV/AIDS Factsheet, 2008). Of the approximately 9 million new cases of TB that occurred in the world in 2007, more than 1 million were associated with HIV co-infection. Approximately 80 percent of patients with both HIV and TB live in sub-Saharan Africa and another 11 percent live in Southeast Asia, meaning that more than 90 percent of the burden of co-infection occurs in just two regions. In 2007, almost a half-million people died of HIV-associated TB (World Health Organization, TB/HIV FACTS 2009, 2009).

While the majority of people affected with HIV and TB co-infection live in developing countries, it is important to know that the problem is not limited to these areas. In the United States in 2005, it was estimated that 9 percent of all TB cases and almost 16 percent of TB cases among people in the 25-to 44-year-old age group occurred in people who were already infected with HIV (Centers for Disease Control, TB and HIV/AIDS Factsheet, 2008). HIV is the greatest threat to meeting TB control goals in countries with high levels of HIV and AIDS.

Over the past 20 years, a great deal of knowledge has been gained about the HIV virus and AIDS. Advances in understanding HIV transmission, improving diagnosis, and treating the infection and its related complications have made an enormous impact on the economically advantaged countries of the developed world. Antiretroviral therapy, a treatment regimen made up of a combination of drugs that are effective in controlling HIV, has greatly reduced complications and death in patients with HIV-related diseases and AIDS. Antiretroviral therapy has transformed HIV/AIDS from a fatal disease into a manageable, chronic condition for patients who can afford treatment and who have access to the combination of drugs. Unfortunately, antiretroviral therapy has had little or no impact throughout developing nations. For the majority of HIV-infected people in Africa, there are no facilities to diagnose HIV and related conditions, no access to antiretroviral therapy, no routine preventive therapies for opportunistic infections that occur when immunity is compromised, and no ability to pay for treatment. For these reasons, the HIV pandemic rages on in poor countries throughout the world and a disease like TB takes full advantage of an impaired immune system.

HIV-infected patients respond as well to anti-TB drugs as HIV-negative patients. There is, however, a higher frequency of complications during TB treatment in HIV-positive patients. Patients who have both TB and HIV are more likely to die than patients who have only one of the diseases. In sub-Saharan Africa, for example, approximately 20 percent to 30 percent of patients with both HIV and smear-positive TB die within 12 months of starting TB treatment, and another 25 percent die during the next 12 months (Dye et al., 2006). There is evidence that delayed TB diagnosis and treatment may compromise the chances of curing TB in HIV-positive patients and untreated TB may accelerate the decline of immune function.

The rapid increase in TB cases associated with the spread of HIV has strained health systems and services in developing nations. Even in countries that have a good DOTS program, high HIV prevalence is associated with increased numbers of TB cases, suggesting that additional strategies may be needed to reduce TB in countries with a high HIV burden. Active case monitoring in high-risk environments, such as prisons and refugee camps, may be an effective way to identify HIV/TB co-infection. Additionally, the use of the anti-TB drug isoniazid for 6 to 12 months significantly reduces an HIV-positive patient's risk of contracting TB, so preventing infection may prove to be an effective strategy of TB control for these patients.

In order to respond to the one-two punch of HIV and TB, countries with high burdens of the diseases are encouraged to implement collaborative TB/HIV activities and related services. Collaborative care means that agencies and health care providers from each disease sector work together to serve patients who have HIV/TB co-infection. In response to high rates of HIV/TB co-infection, the number of countries offering collaborative services increased from just 7 countries in 2003 to 135 countries in 2007. The World Health Organization has identified several essential ways to reduce the HIV/TB epidemic in countries that are the most severely impacted: HIV and TB advocacy efforts must be organized to address both diseases simultaneously; for collaborative programs to be effective, there must be clearly defined roles and responsibilities for HIV and TB advocacy groups to guide activities, mobilize efforts, and manage resources; and HIV and TB groups should each monitor and evaluate collaborative activities and programs to assess the quality, effectiveness, availability, and delivery of services to patients with HIV/TB co-infection.

To decrease the burden of TB in people living with HIV, emphasis on three strategies that begin with the letter *I* is advocated. *Intensified* TB case-finding programs must be established among people with HIV. Programs need to include screening for symptoms and signs of TB in places where there are many HIV-infected people, followed by diagnosis and prompt treatment. Intensified TB case finding increases the chances of survival, improves quality of life, and reduces TB transmission among patients with HIV. *Isoniazid* prevention therapy should be given to people with HIV once it is determined that the patient does not have active TB. Isoniazid is the antibiotic given to people with latent TB infection to prevent its progression to active disease. Using a similar strategy, HIV programs should provide isoniazid therapy for people with HIV to prevent them from contracting TB. Isoniazid prevention therapy can be given in conjunction with antiretroviral drugs. *Infection* control must be ensured in places where people with TB and HIV are crowded together, such as in hospital wards, prisons, or military barracks. These types of facilities must have effective TB control plans in place, including environmental and personal protection measures to reduce transmission.

Conversely, in order to decrease the burden of HIV in patients with TB, several additional strategies are advocated. Since the vast majority of HIV-infected people do not know their HIV status, it is imperative that TB patients be tested for HIV. Knowledge of HIV status gives TB patients an opportunity to receive a continuum of prevention, care, and support for both diseases. Additionally, TB patients should be counseled on ways to prevent HIV, including the promotion of safe and responsible sexual behavior. Patients with active TB and HIV co-infection should be provided with medication to prevent secondary bacterial and parasitic infections. During and after TB treatment, patients with TB and HIV need appropriate care and support for both diseases, and ways to provide antiretroviral therapy to TB patients who are able to have treatment should be in place.

There has been exceptional progress addressing TB/HIV in countries that have implemented collaborative HIV and TB treatment programs, such as

---

Ways to Reduce the Burden of TB among People Living with HIV

HIV care agencies should include three steps that begin with the letter *I* to help tame TB/HIV co-infection:

1. *Intensified* case finding for TB among patients infected with HIV
2. *Isoniazid* antibiotic medication used as preventive therapy
3. *Infection* control

The Stop TB Partnership advocates that these three steps be included as core functions of all HIV treatment services.

Kenya, Rwanda, Malawi, Mozambique, and Tanzania. In Kenya, Malawi, and Rwanda, the percentage of TB patients who were tested for HIV infection greatly increased between 2004 and 2007. In one year, the percentage of TB patients tested for HIV in Mozambique increased from 24 percent to 70 percent, and in Tanzania, the percentage of TB patients who were tested for HIV has increased from 3 percent to 50 percent. About twice as many people living with HIV were screened for TB in 2007 as in 2006, but only a small fraction of the estimated 30 million people living with HIV were put on isoniazid therapy as a measure to prevent TB co-infection (World Health Organization, TB/HIV FACTS 2009). Additionally, since TB infection control measures are not routinely implemented in many HIV service settings, HIV patients may be at risk of acquiring TB while they receive HIV services.

Increased numbers of TB cases resulting from HIV/TB co-infection greatly increase the difficulties associated with TB control and may necessitate the reorganization and decentralization of health care systems in developing countries so that all affected patients can be reached. Increased numbers of workers to record cases and do laboratory work, greater laboratory resources and increased supplies of drugs, and additional hospital facilities to accommodate patients without overcrowding and increasing risk of hospital-born TB infection are required to serve patients in areas with high rates of TB/HIV co-infection. Continued investment in and support of TB control efforts and the need for collaboration between TB and AIDS control programs are vital measures for control of both diseases. HIV and TB occur hand-in-hand—for this reason, AIDS control is an essential element of TB control.

Multidrug-Resistant Tuberculosis

While the spread of HIV infection is contributing to an increasing number of TB cases, drug-resistant TB is making the situation even worse by producing cases that are not responsive to standard treatment. The phenomenon of treatment resistance is not new. Almost as soon as streptomycin was introduced in 1944, the first report of a TB strain that did not respond to the treatment was reported. As a result, treatment with antibiotic combinations was introduced to combat the problem. However, TB that is resistant to more than one first-line anti-TB drug is a more recent problem. The first cases of multidrug-resistant TB were described in the early 1970s, shortly after the introduction of the powerful anti-TB drug rifampin. Multidrug-resistant TB is the result of poorly supervised or incorrectly administered treatment or of initial infection with a TB strain that is already resistant to treatment. As outbreaks of multidrug-resistant TB became increasingly common in 1980s, another dark shadow fell on the hope of worldwide TB control.

Standard TB treatment as recommended by the World Health Organization is successful in 85 percent of patients with TB strains that respond to standard drugs (World Health Organization, Global Tuberculosis Control 2009). Conversely, only 62 percent of patients with drug-resistant cases achieve treatment success (World Health Organization, Anti-Tuberculosis Drug-Resistance in the World, 2008). If first-line treatment is unsuccessful, second-line drugs can treat the infection, but they are more expensive, less accessible, more toxic, and less potent. As early as 1997, an International Union against Tuberculosis and Lung Disease and World Health Organization surveillance project found multidrug-resistant TB in every country it studied, and in 2000, a follow-up report stated that multidrug-resistant TB cases were being found in settings where it had not previously been a problem. Geographical hot spots of multidrug-resistant TB were identified and included areas in Central and Eastern Europe, Russia, Latin America, and China. Not surprisingly, the occurrence of multidrug-resistant TB is highest in countries with poor or nonexistent national TB control programs.

The development and spread of multidrug-resistant TB outpaced worldwide public health efforts to react to it. Determining the best way to respond to multidrug-resistant TB initially caused considerable argument and debate among TB experts worldwide. Some TB control experts argued that, because standard TB control strategies had failed to diagnose and treat drug-susceptible TB, there was no hope that multidrug-resistant cases could be controlled in poor countries. Other experts advocated that short-course therapy based on treatment with isoniazid and rifampin might still be effective in patients with multidrug-resistant TB, although the support of single-drug therapy for multidrug-resistant TB appears to be based more on the cost-effectiveness of this type of treatment rather than on its supposed efficacy in this type of TB.

The debate about whether and how to treat multidrug-resistant TB might have remained a thorny issue if not for the epidemic resurgence of TB in Russia and other parts of the former Soviet Union. The world's first significant outbreak of drug-resistant TB demonstrated that the use of single-drug therapy in multidrug-resistant cases was ineffective and resulted in low cure rates. The resurgence further showed that failure to treat patients with infectious multidrug-resistant TB meant that multidrug-resistant strains of the disease would continue to spread. Since patients with multidrug-resistant TB will not, by definition, respond to the drugs used in the DOTS strategy, another plan to treat this form of TB was needed. Building on the cornerstone of global TB control, enhanced DOTS programs called DOTS-Plus were established to treat multidrug-resistant

TB in places where successful DOTS programs were already in operation. Conceived in Peru in 1998 to control an escalating multidrug-resistant TB problem, DOTS-Plus relies on testing for drug susceptibility and the use of second-line drugs for treatment of drug-resistant cases.

Paul Farmer, a physician and anthropologist who specializes in infectious disease control, was at the center of the effort to convince the world that treatment of multidrug-resistant TB was both possible and necessary. With the goal of transforming health care on a global scale, in 1987 Farmer helped to found a nonprofit organization called Partners in Health (PIH). Ultimately, PIH would help to define new treatment approaches for multidrug-resistant TB. Along with its sister organizations in Peru and Russia, PIH led a world-wide effort to institute effective treatment regimens to combat multidrug-resistant TB. They continue to advocate for public health services and second-line antibiotic treatment to curb TB transmission in the most poverty-stricken areas of the world.

The fight against multidrug-resistant strains of TB began in 1996, when an epidemic of multidrug-resistant TB was discovered in Lima, Peru. The treatment arsenal included the use of second-line anti-TB drugs, a previously unheard of strategy in developing nations, and patient support measures. To encourage treatment adherence, people from the community were trained and hired to help patients get through the long and arduous course of treatment needed for multidrug-resistant TB. Because the drugs needed to treat multidrug-resistant TB are both expensive and difficult to obtain, the World Health Organization initially considered the treatment of multidrug-resistant TB impractical and un-affordable. However, Farmer, PIH, and Peruvian agencies created a compelling argument in favor of treating multidrug-resistant TB in developing countries by achieving an astonishing 83 percent cure rate with their initial attempt at a comprehensive treatment approach in Peru. As a result, in 2002, the World Health Organization began approving plans to treat multidrug-resistant TB on a country-by-country basis. Four years later, new guidelines for treating multidrug-resistant TB and a plan to increase the number of patients receiving treatment were initiated, indicating that treating multidrug-resistant TB was now considered to be both realistic and crucial to achieving global TB control.

Multidrug-resistant TB treatment guidelines were also influenced by the success of PIH treatment strategies that were used in Siberia, Russia. PIH began working in Siberia in 1998 to expand the drug-resistant TB treatment model that was developed in Peru. The organization renovated TB hospitals, trained medical personnel, and distributed educational materials throughout the former Soviet Union. By February 2005, more than 1,500 TB and multidrug-resistant TB patients had received treatment and support from PIH. The first group of multidrug-resistant patients achieved an amazing 78 percent cure rate. The efforts of Paul Farmer and PIH have established that treating multidrug-resistant TB is effective and feasible, demonstrating the need for continued expansion of DOTS-Plus programs into the multidrug-resistant hot spots. Since improved diagnosis and adequate treatment of TB that responds to first-line drugs results in the creation of fewer drug-resistant TB bacteria and fewer cases of multidrug-resistant TB, treatment of drug-susceptible cases with the right anti-TB drugs as quickly as possible and for as long as necessary remains the bedrock of all TB control. However, when multidrug-resistant TB is identified, second-line drugs can and should be used to treat this escalating TB problem.

THE MAJOR TARGETS OF TUBERCULOSIS CONTROL

Four major objectives have been established to make the goal of global TB control a reality: (1) by 2015, the rate of occurrence of new cases of TB should be declining; (2) by 2015, the level of TB in the global population and deaths due to it should be half of what they were in 1990; (3) at least 70 percent of new smear-positive TB cases should be detected and treated in a DOTS program; and (4) treatment of new smear-positive cases should be successful at least 85 percent of the time. So, where does global TB control stand? World Health Organization data from 2009 suggest that the rate of occurrence of new cases of TB has been falling since 2004, but global decline is very slow. The five countries with the highest total number of TB cases in 2007 were India, China, Indonesia, Nigeria, and South Africa. Of new TB cases reported, about 15 percent occurred in people who were also HIV-positive, with most of these HIV-positive cases occurring in Africa and a smaller number in Southeast Asia. It is estimated that TB prevalence and death rates will be cut in half in some regions of the world by the target date, but the goal will not be achieved for the world as a whole. In 2007, the rate of case detection was a little lower than what was hoped, but the goal of successfully treating 85 percent of the people who have TB was reached in 2006. It is apparent that international efforts have made some progress toward reaching the long-term goals set for TB control, but the question remains—what else can be done to eliminate this killer of the ages?

8

Tuberculosis and the Future

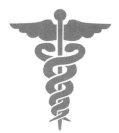

I n spite of the progress that has been made toward controlling the occurrence and spread of TB, it remains the second leading cause of death from infectious disease in the world. The global burden of TB is falling slowly, and in at least some of the regions delineated by the World Health Organization, it appears that global targets for reducing the number of TB cases and deaths will be reached. Increasing numbers of individuals with TB have access to high-quality anti-TB treatment and related interventions, such as antiretroviral therapy for HIV co-infection. In spite of this fact, it is estimated that more than one-third of new TB cases are not being treated in a DOTS program, and up to 96 percent of new cases caused by multidrug-resistant strains are not being diagnosed and treated according to international guidelines. Additionally, the majority of people who are both HIV-positive and have TB are not aware of their HIV status, and the majority of HIV-positive TB patients who do know their HIV status do not have access to antiretroviral therapy (World Health Organization, 2009). The preponderance of TB is concentrated in specific countries and regions of the world. Inadequate local resources to control TB in developing countries, poverty, the global epidemic of HIV, and increased multidrug-resistant cases are among the root causes of the continuing global TB crisis. Internationally, TB is very much alive—thriving on the social, economic, and political chaos that defines

Tuberculosis in Countries

The 22 countries shown on the map accounts for 80% of the TB cases in the world

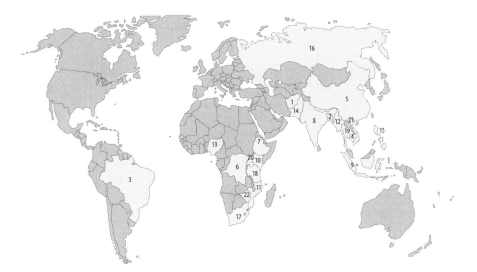

The numbers on this map correspond to the alphabetical listing of the country.

ALPHABETICAL

1. Afghanistan
2. Bangladesh
3. Brazil
4. Cambodia
5. China
6. Democratic Republic of Congo
7. Ethiopia
8. India
9. Indonesia
10. Kenya
11. Mozambique
12. Myanmar
13. Nigeria
14. Pakistan
15. Philippines
16. Russian Federation
17. South Africa
18. United Republic of Tanzania
19. Thailand
20. Uganda
21. Viet Nam
22. Zimbabwe

RANK BY BURDEN

1. India
2. China
3. Indonesia
4. Nigeria
5. South Africa
6. Bangladesh
7. Ethiopia
8. Pakistan
9. Philippines
10. Democratic Republic of Congo
11. Russian Federation
12. Viet Nam
13. Kenya
14. Brazil
15. United Republic of Tanzania
16. Uganda
17. Zimbabwe
18. Thailand
19. Mozambique
20. Myanmar
21. Cambodia
22. Afghanistan

A map of the 22 countries that account for 80 percent of the TB cases in the world (World Health Organization, Global Tuberculosis Control 2009). India currently bears the greatest global burden of TB. Courtesy of the Stop TB Partnership and the World Health Organization, http://www.stoptb.org/countries/.

the environment of many developing nations. Controlling and eliminating TB will require continued worldwide effort on several fronts.

FUTURE DRUG TREATMENTS FOR TUBERCULOSIS

Although antibiotic drugs that cure TB have been available for many years, TB is still one of the leading causes of infectious disease in the world. Part of reason for the gap between effective use of anti-TB drugs and control of the disease is related to the duration and complexity of the treatment regimen that is necessary to produce a cure. The course of therapy that is currently available to patients with TB requires that they take four different antibiotics for two months, followed by continued rifampin and isoniazid for an additional four months. Some of the drugs need to be taken after eating, while others are supposed to be taken on an empty stomach. They can cause unpleasant side effects and produce liver toxicity. In other words, even though treatments to cure TB are available and relatively inexpensive, the process of being cured is long and difficult. When the burden of TB treatment interferes with its completion and success, the patient may remain ill, may continue to be infectious, and may develop a multidrug-resistant strain of TB that is ultimately even more difficult to treat.

A primary goal of anti-TB drug development is the discovery of new treatments that will shorten the length of treatment, are compatible with antiretroviral therapy for patients who have HIV/TB co-infection, and are effective against multidrug-resistant strains and latent TB infection. Additionally, medications that are already in existence are being re-evaluated for their potential efficacy in fighting TB. For example, the flouroquinolone wide-spectrum antibiotics, which are already so useful in the treatment of multidrug-resistant TB, are being tested in clinical trials to determine if they have a potential to shorten first-line anti-TB therapy.

New drug development proceeds in stages until clinical tests determine that a new product is safe and effective for use in humans. Deliberate efforts are being made to identify and develop specific drugs that are active against M. *tuberculosis* bacteria by screening large numbers of new compounds to determine how effective they are at stopping actively reproducing bacteria. If a new compound is found that can stop M. *tuberculosis* from reproducing, further investigation is undertaken to discover how it works and to guide the drug development process. Because current treatments are not very effective against multidrug-resistant TB, investigational new drugs are evaluated in patients with multidrug-resistant forms of disease to gauge their strength. This means that new anti-TB drugs can be preliminarily tested on fewer patients and small-scale success can pave the way for testing in larger trials with more patients.

Evaluating new drugs for TB treatment is a difficult undertaking because there are no good ways to measure an early prediction of cure or relapse. In addition, fear of provoking the development of resistance to a new drug limits the testing of single treatments to a very short period of time, meaning that the full effect of a new drug may not even have a chance to develop. In spite of these limitations, the hunt-and-peck method of discovering new anti-TB drugs has uncovered some promising candidates that appear to offer hope for treating TB and multidrug-resistant TB in the future.

Diarylquinoline is a new drug that is in development for the fight against TB. With a mechanism of activity that is different from other antibiotic drugs, diarylquinoline has demonstrated that it can inhibit both drug-susceptible and drug-resistant TB bacteria in pure cultures, and it appears to be able to kill latent bacteria as well. When used in combination with a five-drug, second-line drug treatment regimen, combination diarylquinoline treatment had tolerable side effects; reduced the time needed to produce a negative sputum culture in patients with newly diagnosed, sputum-positive, multidrug-resistant TB; and increased the proportion of patients with negative sputum cultures. While only in an early stage of development, diarylquinoline appears to offer some hope that a drug that works differently from the standard anti-TB treatments may be a future tool in the war against TB.

Other innovative ways to use drugs to control TB are also being studied to increase the number of anti-TB therapies. Two antibiotics that are already used for treating other bacterial infections were recently shown to have a potential for treating extensively drug-resistant TB, the most deadly form of the infection, when they are used in combination therapy. Working as partners, one of the antibiotics inhibits a bacterial enzyme that normally shields TB bacteria; then, while the TB bacteria are not shielded by the enzyme protector, the second antibiotic can move in and kill it. In a laboratory culture, the dual treatment inhibited the growth of drug-susceptible laboratory TB strains, as well as extensively drug-resistant strains isolated from TB patients. While the idea of using an enzyme-inhibiting antibiotic in tandem with another antibiotic is not new, thorough investigation to find the ideal combination of drugs may have finally paid off against extensively drug-resistant TB.

Although only a laboratory concept to date, if a combination treatment such as this one proves to be effective in humans, TB treatment could be simplified to just two drugs that would work against drug-susceptible, multidrug-resistant, and extensively drug-resistant TB strains. An easy, two-drug regimen that is effective against all TB strains could greatly simplify the treatment process, encourage better treatment adherence, and enhance outcomes. Plans are being made to launch two small studies of the combination therapy in humans in South Korea and South Africa. If the small-scale studies are successful and funding is available, additional studies involving larger numbers of patients will be conducted in South Africa because of the disproportionately high number of extensively drug-resistant TB cases there—in some areas of South Africa, one in four TB cases is extensively drug-resistant.

With the coming of age of genome sequencing in molecular biology, specific genes have been identified as potential targets for the development of new anti-TB drugs. The genome of an organism is its hereditary information encoded in deoxyribonucleic acid (DNA). DNA is a nucleic acid that contains the genetic instructions used in the development and functioning of all known living organisms. The genome of an organism is a complete genetic sequence; genome sequencing is a laboratory process that determines the complete DNA sequence of an organism's genome at a single time. The genome sequencing of a prototype *M. tuberculosis* strain was finished in 1998, and sequencing of other *M. tuberculosis* subspecies and other mycobacterial species have been achieved or are under way. Special genetic targets that are essential for the growth of *M. tuberculosis*, but which do not exist or are significantly different in humans, have been identified as new targets for anti-TB drugs. It appears that about 15 percent of *M. tuberculosis* genes are needed for its optimal growth; as a result, these genes have become very attractive targets for new anti-TB drugs.

Genome-sequencing strategies have also been used to gain an understanding of the cellular mechanisms that enable *M. tuberculosis* to become latent. How do the bacteria essentially shut down—stopping reproduction but remaining viable and capable of reactivating? In laboratory models that use nutrient starvation to mimic TB bacteria in a latent state, hundreds of genes that are stimulated during starvation have been identified. Valuable insights into the activity of bacteria-killing compounds that act against dormant tubercle bacilli have been gained through the use of these genetic models. A full course of TB treatment takes many months because latent TB bacteria may reactivate and cause the patient to become sick and infectious again. If genome sequencing can clarify the phenomenon of latency in TB bacteria, it may lead to the development of drugs that can specifically target latent bacteria. In the future, therapies that act against latent TB bacteria may be able to shorten the length of TB treatment, making it easier for patients to complete the whole course of therapy, thus reducing the risk of relapse and the potential development of multidrug-resistant disease strains. It is hoped that the development of new drugs through new technologies or the use of old drugs in new ways will help bring the worldwide TB crisis to a halt.

FUTURE DIRECTIONS IN DIAGNOSTICS

The current strategy of TB control relies on treating patients who have already been diagnosed with active disease. In 2007, 99 percent of TB case reports were made in association with DOTS programs. It is estimated that 63 percent of new smear-positive cases of TB were detected and treated in DOTS programs, still a little short of the 70 percent target goal that was first hoped to be realized in 2000 (World Health Organization, Global Tuberculosis Control 2009). New drugs to control TB make up only half of a comprehensive TB control strategy—the future of TB control also depends on the ability to rapidly, cheaply, and accurately detect and diagnose the disease in patients who live in every corner of the world. Research to improve the future of TB control must include a focus on improving the ability to diagnose the disease. In most countries, TB diagnosis is still based on results obtained from the microscopic examination of sputum to find acid-fast bacteria, a method that was developed 120 years ago. Although the smear technique is relatively inexpensive and quick, it accurately identifies only 40 percent to 60 percent of people who actually have TB because of its tendency to give false negative results; accuracy of sputum microscopy decreases to 20 percent for people who have HIV co-infection.

False negative results mean that people who actually have TB are not reaping the benefits of early diagnosis and treatment, leaving additional numbers of people at risk of exposure to infection. Sputum culture is much more accurate at identifying TB, but it takes several weeks to obtain results because the bacteria must grow under laboratory conditions to make a diagnosis. Molecular biological methods of detection are accurate and rapid, but they are expensive and require the use of advanced technology. Furthermore, all these methods rely on the identification of active TB in the sputum, which means that, by the time the disease is diagnosed, the patient is already infectious; latent or early TB cannot be detected at all. Because of these limitations, TB diagnosis is still supported by the use of skin testing and chest x-ray.

New diagnostic TB tests that are based on the identification of antigens, any substance that is foreign to the body and evokes an immune response, are being investigated. The development of point-of-care diagnostic tests based on mycobacterial antigens and other proteins that are found in the genes of M. *tuberculosis* is one of the future directions of TB diagnostics. New diagnostic tests to identify TB must be cost effective, easy to use in all health care systems, and not dependent on the availability of sophisticated laboratory services. New tests for TB diagnosis also need to be able to perform equally well in individuals with or without HIV infection, should discriminate between an immune response produced by vaccination or real M. *tuberculosis* infection, and should enable accurate and timely detection of TB cases.

THE FUTURE OF TUBERCULOSIS VACCINATION

The BCG vaccine was introduced in 1921, and since that time it has remained essentially unchanged. It is widely used in developing countries to protect children from the ravages of TB, although its effectiveness in preventing pulmonary TB in adults and its preventive powers over time are questionable. In any case, the unacceptably high incidence of TB around the world and the increase of multidrug-resistant TB strains are evidence that better measures of TB prevention are needed to control the spread of the disease.

Current strategies for developing new vaccines are either directed at improving the BCG vaccine for preventive purposes or developing a new post-exposure vaccine to prevent latent TB infection from reactivating. It has been estimated that a vaccine that could effectively prevent the development of infection after a person has been exposed to TB could prevent 30 percent to 40 percent of TB cases. In recent years, attempts have also been made to improve pre-exposure vaccines by developing live vaccine alternatives and novel booster vaccines. In the future, booster doses may be used either to strengthen the immunity of the BCG vaccine to prevent primary disease or to strengthen immunity in individuals with latent infection for prevention of reactivation. These approaches to TB vaccine development have been greatly enriched by the availability of the genome sequence.

An experimental vaccine called MVA85A, the first new TB vaccine to be offered in 80 years, is ready to begin a more advanced stage of development. The new vaccine, which is designed to be given alongside the current BCG vaccine, works by stimulating T cells in the immune system to produce a stronger response to the BCG vaccine. In the first series of tests, administered in 2007, the new vaccine was shown to be safe and scientists are now ready to test its effectiveness in infants in South Africa. If the next tests are successful, it is hoped that a new vaccine to boost the success of the BCG vaccine could be available by 2016.

New vaccination strategies will probably be necessary to cover the varying needs that exist within different populations around the world. The use of vaccination as a primary TB prevention plan will require special consideration of places where many individuals have already been vaccinated with the BCG vaccine or where environmental exposure to mycobacteria has already primed the immune system. Additionally, the needs of patients with HIV infection and/or those who have latent TB infection will also need to be taken into account.

WORLDWIDE TUBERCULOSIS: THE GLOBAL EFFORT

World Tuberculosis Day is observed annually on the 24th of March, the anniversary of the day Robert Koch announced the discovery of M. *Tuberculosis*, the microorganism that causes TB. Events associated with the anniversary are designed to increase public awareness of the prevalence of TB in many places around the world and to draw attention to the horrifying consequences it still produces. The reality that TB remains a global crisis is eloquently summed up in the slogan from World Tuberculosis Day 2007—"TB Anywhere Is TB Everywhere." Global TB control and eradication is, by necessity, the responsibility of every country in the world regardless of individual national TB burdens.

Worldwide TB incidence has declined since 2004, but only by about 1 percent annually. The relationship between HIV and TB has thoroughly complicated the prognosis for both diseases, especially in sub-Saharan Africa. Additionally, the increase in cases of multidrug-resistant TB and extensively multidrug-resistant strains, especially in Eastern Europe, threaten the ability to successfully treat the disease and may cause increased rates of TB death. What steps can be taken to manage the current burden of global TB and how can future cases be prevented in all parts of the world?

The World Health Organization, the U.S. Centers for Disease Control and Prevention, and various partner agencies are taking steps to help stop the spread of TB worldwide. Even though the original goals set forth by the Stop TB Partnership will not be met on schedule, the strategy remains sound. Steps to improve TB control activities while dealing with the spread of TB/HIV co-infection and multidrug-resistant TB serve as the backbone of the plan. The components of the Stop TB Partnership strategy builds on the success of DOTS, the World Health Organization initiative that has guided TB treatment for over 22 million patients.

Beyond improved prevention, diagnosis, and treatment of TB, complementary programs must also address the social and environmental factors that increase the

---

The Basic Principles of the Stop TB Partnership

1. Pursue high-quality DOTS expansion and enhancement into the most remote regions to make high-quality services widely available to all who need them, including the poorest and most vulnerable
2. Address TB/HIV, multidrug-resistant TB, and other challenges
3. Strengthen health systems so national TB control programs can contribute to overall TB control strategies including financing, planning, and management
4. Engage all care providers, including health care workers from public, private, corporate, and voluntary sources, to reach all patients
5. Empower people with TB and their communities through networks to mobilize society and to ensure political support to maintain long-term TB control programs
6. Enable and promote research to improve TB control practices through new diagnostics, drugs, and vaccines

risk of developing TB. Poverty and the factors associated with it—homelessness, political unrest, overcrowded living conditions, poor nutrition, and lack of access to medical care—remain the ever-present contributors to TB incidence. Programs that create a collaborative approach to improve the human condition from every vantage point are needed to stop TB. International concerns, governments, corporations, private foundations, social service workers, health care providers, and individuals will need to combine their resources and skills to accomplish the seemingly impossible task of finally ridding the world of the burden of TB.

ELIMINATING TUBERCULOSIS IN THE UNITED STATES

According to the most recent Centers for Disease Control and Prevention data that are available, the lowest rate of TB ever recorded in the United States since national TB reporting began in 1953 was reported in 2007 (Centers for Disease Control, Trends in Tuberculosis—United States, 2007, 2008). The resurgence of TB in the 1980s caused renewed national, state, and local response and the success of this cohesive effort has demonstrated that TB control can be achieved. The goal of eliminating TB in the United States was rekindled by this success and it remains very much alive. However, in spite of historically low rates of TB and an Institute of Medicine study published in 2000 that confirmed that TB could indeed be eliminated, at the present rate of decline, it would take more than 70 years to fully stamp out TB in the United States.

Since seven more decades of TB in the United States are not considered an acceptable timeline, a comprehensive plan to speed up the rate of decline and make TB elimination a more readily reachable goal has been developed. The plan includes components that are designed to fine-tune TB control measures to better identify high-risk populations in light of declining incidence in general. It provides increased testing for people who are more likely to be exposed to or infected by TB, as well as more aggressive identification and treatment of latent TB infection. Additionally, national TB control plans are calling for the development of new tools to improve diagnosis, treatment, and prevention of the disease, mobilization of public support, and increased involvement in global TB control efforts.

The high rate of TB among foreign-born people living in the United States and among racial and ethnic minorities indicates that efforts to control TB need to be concentrated in these populations. Delays in detecting and reporting cases, insufficient protection for persons who are commonly in contact with infectious TB patients, and inadequate prevention and response to TB outbreaks are among the factors that hinder progress toward eradication of the disease. Prior experience has demonstrated that during times of declining TB incidence, it is imperative to maintain clinical and public health capabilities. Throughout history,

TB has made many comebacks—the goal of complete eradication in the United States demands continuing vigilance and effort. The United States cannot afford to let its guard down until TB is eliminated in all parts of the world.

The increased burden of HIV and TB co-infection is a threat to TB control in both the United States and on a global level. In response to the publication of a recent report from the Center for Global Health Policy entitled *Deadly Duo: The Synergy Between HIV/AIDS and Tuberculosis*, on June 25, 2009, leading disease experts called on President Barack Obama and the U.S. Congress. At a congressional briefing, they emphasized the need for strong leadership from the United States in response to the threat from HIV/TB co-infection and called for significant new funding for TB and HIV treatment, prevention, and research. According to the report, future White House actions to prevent a global health catastrophe should include a Presidential Initiative on Tuberculosis to ensure an all-encompassing response to the threat posed by HIV/TB co-infection. Congress was encouraged to ensure that the amount of funding for TB control is equal to the seriousness of the co-infection epidemic by doubling spending for basic TB research and finding more effective anti-TB drugs. HIV agencies were delegated the responsibility for ensuring that HIV patients are screened for TB and either treated for the disease or given preventive therapy in settings with good infection control measures. Continued improvement of the quality of antiretroviral therapy and access to it for all HIV patients is an essential piece of the fight against HIV/TB co-infection.

Eliminating TB in the United States will require the cooperation of professionals from diverse areas of health science and society. Although the public health sector will continue to play a critical role in the planning, coordination, and evaluation of the effort to stamp out TB, the traditional public health model of TB control may no longer be the best approach in the United States. Similar to global efforts, the final push for TB eradication in the United States will require the hard work of many. Private-sector clinicians, immigration workers, the prison

---

The Basic Principles of TB Control in the United States

1. Early and accurate detection, diagnosis, and reporting of cases to the appropriate public health agency
2. Identification and evaluation of people who have had contact with people who have infectious TB or who are at high risk of developing infection
3. Identification of and effective treatment for people with latent TB
4. Identification of high-risk settings (e.g., prisons, nursing homes) and the use of effective infection control measures in these environments

The Face of Tuberculosis Now

Throughout history, the face of TB has changed with the times. The ancient Egyptians, the workers of the Industrial Revolution, the Romantic poets, racial minorities in the United States, and the poor who live in developing counties are among those who have worn the mask of TB. What does TB look like today? Thembi Ngubane, a South African health activist, was 19 years old when she began keeping an audio diary to chronicle her experience living with HIV/AIDS. The HIV virus infects nearly one-third of young South African women, yet the stigma against it remains so strong that many people are too scared to even tell their family and friends they have it. U.S. National Public Radio began to air her tapes in a production called *Radio Diaries* in April 2006, on her 21st birthday. She began her story by reciting what she called her "HIV Prayer": "Hello HIV, you trespasser. You are in my body, you have to obey the rules. You have to respect me and if you don't hurt me, I won't hurt you. You mind your business and I will mind mine and I will give you a ticket when your time comes." Millions of radio listeners around the world learned about the AIDS epidemic in South Africa through Ngubane and they got to know her. They contributed money to her family and helped them purchase their own house in the township of Khayelitsha. She was invited on a tour of the United States, where she met former President Bill Clinton and spoke to students, lawmakers, doctors, and celebrities about her struggles living with AIDS. But ultimately, the story that Ngubane told was the tale of the relationship between AIDS and TB. In June 2009, at the age of 24, Ngubane died—not from AIDS, as might have been expected, but from multidrug-resistant TB, the frequent co-conspirator of AIDS. When the immune response is compromised by HIV/AIDS, multidrug-resistant TB does not obey any rules, and all too frequently it becomes a death sentence. Ngubane leaves behind her four-year-old daughter, Onwabo, her partner, her mother, two sisters, and a brother.

system, community health centers, HIV agencies, hospitals, educators, and the pharmaceutical industry must all be involved in the effort. The elimination of TB in the United States must proceed from a global perspective. TB anywhere is TB everywhere—the key to finally doing away with TB in the United States ultimately depends on the success of national and international efforts to contain TB in every part of the world.

TUBERCULOSIS DOES NOT GET THE LAST WORD...

TB has been a plague on the health and well-being of people throughout the ages. From antiquity to the present day, TB has staked its claim, stalked its victims, and stolen their youth, their vitality, and their lives. Although not un-known among kings, the destitute and downtrodden are both the historical and contemporary victims of the M. *tuberculosis* bacteria, the germ that keeps on killing. The effort to ultimately eradicate TB must occur at every level of soci-ety—local, regional, national, and global—and it will require an international standard of care for all TB patients.

Although ideal conditions for the survival of TB are still a reality in many parts of the world, some tools to eliminate it already exist and others must be developed through a collaborative global effort. TB/HIV co-infection, multidrug-resistant and extensively drug-resistant strains, weak health care systems in many developing nations, and global poverty are factors that demand the attention of those charged with leading the effort to control TB. Laboratories and clinicians around the world must follow the best diagnostic, reporting, and case manage-ment practices that are available, and they must have the tools to do so. In ad-dition, new treatments and diagnostic techniques must be developed to improve worldwide TB outcomes. New anti-TB drugs that shorten treatment duration and simplify care would inevitably improve a patient's ability to complete therapy and effect a cure. And finally, to echo the sentiments advanced by René Jules Dubos many years ago, TB will ultimately be surmounted through consideration of the ecological, economic, political, and cultural factors that exist in local surround-ings where the disease still flourishes. The hope for a world free of TB begins with the cure of an individual patient.

Tuberculosis Timeline

3000 B.C.E.	Physical deformities characteristic of TB in the spine portrayed in the drawings, pottery, and statues of ancient Egypt
460–375 B.C.E.	Hippocrates, called the father of medicine, believes TB is caused by growths in the lungs, which he calls "tubercula"
Second century C.E.	Aretæus notes that a specific type of person (pale with a slender, weak body) is more prone to TB
162 C.E.	Galen recognizes many forms of TB and believes that it can be spread from person to person
To the mid-19th century	Bloodletting is used to treat various illnesses including TB
1300–1600	The European Renaissance; TB occurs in Europe but not as commonly as in previous eras
1620	Half of the Pilgrims who reach the Plymouth, Massachusetts, die during the first winter (no direct evidence of TB as the cause)

1623	Shakespeare describes scrofula and the ritual of the royal touch to cure it in *Macbeth*
1643	King Louis XIII of France dies of TB at the age of 42
1674	Antonie van Leeuwenhoek uses the microscope lens he invented to become the first person to see a microorganism
1711	Samuel Johnson is touched by Queen Anne in a healing ritual to cure scrofula
1720	Benjamin Marten speculates that TB may be caused by "wonderfully minute living creatures"
1775–1783	The American Revolutionary War; TB is a well-established disease in the colonies
Late 18th and early 19th centuries	Industrial Revolution in Europe; a time of vast increase in the incidence of TB
1800	Child labor becomes commonplace in the factories of England, increasing the risk of contracting TB
1800–1850	TB is the deadliest disease in America, responsible for one in five deaths
1816	René Théophile Hyacinthe Laënnec invents the first stethoscope, which helps physicians assess respiratory illnesses including TB
1821	John Keats dies of TB
1825	Maria and Elizabeth Brontë die of TB
1839	Tuberculosis is suggested as the generic term to describe all forms of phthisis
1840s	Iodine solution becomes a popular TB remedy
1840s–1880s	TB encourages migration to the American West for people seeking climates conducive to better health
1847–1849	Emily, Anne, and Branwell Brontë die of TB
Mid-1800s	Incidence of TB in America reaches its peak
1850	Incidence of TB in Europe reaches its peak
1850s	Cod-liver oil gains favor as a TB treatment

1853	*La Traviata*, by Giuseppe Verdi, premieres; the plot features a heroine who dies of TB
1855	Charlotte Brontë dies of TB and complications of pregnancy
1859	The first sanatorium specifically devoted to the treatment of lung diseases is opened in Germany by Dr. Hermann Brehmer
1860s	Louis Pasteur is the first to show that microorganisms, such as bacteria, cause many diseases
1865	Jean Antoine Villemin begins laboratory experiments to evaluate TB transmission in animals
1882	Robert Koch, a German microbiologist, presents irrefutable evidence that TB is caused by M. *tuberculosis*
1884	Edward Livingston Trudeau establishes the first TB sanatorium in the United States in Saranac Lake, New York
1885	Edvard Munch paints *The Sick Child*, portraying his sister's death from TB
1890–1920	Public health crusades against tenement housing, sweatshops, child labor, public spitting and coughing, and unpasteurized milk are mounted in the United States to fight the spread of TB
1894	Carlo Forliani introduces artificial pneumothorax for the treatment of TB
1895	Wilhelm Konrad von Röntgen discovers x-ray
1896	*La Bohème*, by Giacomo Puccini, premieres; the plot features a heroine who dies of TB
1900	Robert Koch discovers tuberculin
1904	The first nationwide voluntary health organization focused on conquering a specific disease, the National Association for the Study and Prevention of Tuberculosis, is founded
1905	Robert Koch is awarded the Nobel Prize in Medicine

1907	Clemens Freiherr Baron von Pirquet is the first to use tuberculin skin testing in humans
1907	The first American Christmas Seal campaign is mounted to raise money for TB
1920s	The use of chest x-rays to help diagnose and assess TB is well established
1920s	African Americans are affected by TB more than any other single group in the United States
1921	Léon Charles Albert Calmette and Camille Guérin administer the Bacillus Calmette-Guérin (BCG) vaccine to a human being for the first time
1925	There are 536 sanatoria with 673,338 beds in operation in the United States
1924	*The Magic Mountain*, by Thomas Mann, is published; the novel is set in a sanatorium and all the characters suffer from TB
Late 1920s	TB skin testing is common in the United States
1928	The League of Nations certifies that the BCG vaccine is safe for use in humans
1940	Selman Waksman isolates the first antibiotic that effectively inhibits the growth of TB bacteria; it is too toxic for use in humans
1942	The term *antibiotic* is coined by Selman Waksman
1943	Selman Waksman discovers streptomycin
1944	The first dose of streptomycin is given to a patient who is critically ill with TB
1947	Mass chest x-ray screening programs are initiated in the United States
1950s	U.S. public health officials think that infectious disease and TB are no longer problems because antibiotics can cure them
1952	Selman Waksman is awarded the Nobel Prize

1952	Isoniazid is discovered
1954	Pyrazinamide is discovered
1960s–1970s	New epidemics of old infectious diseases occur
1960s–1970s	More than 30 new infectious diseases are discovered
1962	Ethambutol is discovered
1963	Rifampin is discovered, and short-course TB treatment is launched
Early 1970s	The first cases of multidrug-resistant TB are described
1970s	TB is rare in the Soviet Union
1975–1976	First signs of a mounting TB epidemic in New York City
1979	Start of the TB epidemic in New York City
1980s	The beginning of worldwide TB resurgence; the end of the steady decline in global TB that began with the advent of antibiotic treatment
1984–1997	In London, rates of overcrowding increase by 40 percent and contribute to increasing TB occurrence
1985–1992	20 percent increase in the rate of TB in the United States
1987	Paul Farmer helps found a nonprofit organization called Partners in Health to improve global health care, including the treatment of multidrug-resistant TB
1988	Rate of TB decline in London levels off
1990s	Directly observed therapy, short-course (DOTS) program is launched by the World Health Organization
1990s	Prevalence of TB in Russia triples; many cases are resistant to at least one first-line treatment
1991	Collapse of the Soviet Union brings changing social conditions that contribute to increased rates of TB
1993	Well-funded DOTS program is initiated in New York City
1993	Rate of TB in New York City begins to decline

1993	World Health Organization declares a "global health emergency" in response to increases in the incidence of TB in developing countries
1993–2003	44 percent decline in TB incidence in the United States
Mid-1990s	International Committee of the Red Cross reveals that there are dangerous levels of TB infection in Russian prisons
Mid-1990s	Red Cross and Médecins Sans Frontières (Doctors without Borders) begin TB control programs in Russian prisons
1996	Epidemic multidrug-resistant TB in Lima, Peru
1996	*Rent,* a stage musical inspired by the story told in *La Bohème,* opens on Broadway
1997	Multidrug-resistant TB is in every country surveyed by the International Union against Tuberculosis and Lung Disease and the World Health Organization
1998	One in 10 Russian prisoners suffer from active TB; an estimated 20,000 have multidrug-resistant strains
1998	DOTS-Plus program is launched for the treatment of multidrug-resistant TB
1998	Genome sequencing of the prototype strain M. *tuberculosis* is finished
2000	Stop TB Partnership is established
2000	Multidrug-resistant TB cases found in settings where it had not previously been found
2001	*Moulin Rouge!,* a movie inspired by the plot of *La Traviata,* premieres
2002	The World Health Organization begins approving plans to treat multidrug-resistant TB according to the model developed by Partners in Health
2003	Seven countries offer collaborative TB/HIV activities in response to high rates of HIV/TB co-infection

2005	9 percent of all TB cases in the United States are associated with HIV co-infection
2006	The World Health Organization initiates new guidelines for treating multidrug-resistant TB and presents a plan to increase the number of patients treated
2007	99 percent of TB case reports are made in association with DOTS programs
2007	135 countries offer collaborative TB/HIV activities in response to high rates of HIV/TB co-infection
2007	The United States records its lowest rate of TB ever
2007	The TB rate is 9.7 percent higher for foreign-born people living in the United States than for people born in the United States
2007	More than 1 million of the approximately 9 million new cases of TB in the world are associated with HIV co-infection
2007	Almost half a million people die of HIV-associated TB
2009	Call for Presidential Initiative on Tuberculosis to ensure an all-encompassing response to the threat posed by HIV/TB co-infection
2009	South African AIDS activist Thembi Ngubane dies of multidrug-resistant TB

Glossary

Acid-fast bacteria: bacteria that are not decolorized by acids after staining; an identifying characteristic of *Mycobacterium*

Activated macrophage: a mature macrophage whose ability to destroy microbes or other cells has been enhanced because of stimulation by the immune system

Aerobic: living, active, or occurring only when oxygen is present

Alveoli: small air sacs in the lungs

Animalculae: the word coined by Benjamin Marten to describe microorganisms that he observed during early microbiology experiments

Antibiotic: a powerful drug that fights bacterial infections by either killing or preventing infection-causing bacteria from reproducing

Antigens: any substance that is foreign to the body that evokes an immune response

Antiretroviral drugs: medications for the treatment of infection caused by retroviruses, primarily HIV/AIDS

Artificial pneumothorax: surgically induced collapse of the lung

Bacillus Calmette-Guérin (BCG): the vaccine used in developing countries to reduce the most severe consequences of TB in infants and children

Bacteria: round, spiral, or rod-shaped single-celled microorganisms that typically live in soil, water, organic matter, or the bodies of plants and animals; some types are capable of causing disease, while others are harmless or even beneficial

B.C.E.: Before the Common Era

Bovine: relating to cows or oxen

Caseous necrosis: the soft, cheese-like material in the central part of a tubercle lesion

C.E.: the Common Era

Consumption: the biblical name for tuberculosis; the term refers to the wasting away of the body

Culture test: the definitive diagnostic test for TB; a sputum sample is incubated and the bacteria are allowed to grow to permit identification

Directly observed therapy, short-course (DOTS) program: a plan to ensure worldwide access to trained medical personnel and antibiotic agents for all people with TB

DNA (deoxyribonucleic acid): a nucleic acid that contains the genetic instructions used in the development and functioning of all known living organisms

Ethambutal: one of the four first-line anti-TB antibiotics

Extensively drug-resistant TB: a form of tuberculosis that is resistant to at least two first-line anti-TB drugs, any fluoroquinolone, and at least one of three injectable second-line drugs used for treatment

Extra-pulmonary TB: tuberculosis infection that is transported from damaged lung tissue to other parts of the body (e.g., kidney, spine, brain) through the bloodstream; it is usually not contagious

Fluoroquinolone: a relatively new family of synthetic broad-spectrum antibiotics that are used to treat multidrug-resistant TB

Fluoroscope: an imaging technique commonly used to obtain real-time moving images of the internal structures of a patient

Genome: the hereditary information of an organism encoded in its DNA

Genome sequencing: a laboratory process that determines the complete DNA sequence of an organism's genome at a single time

HIV/AIDS: human immunodeficiency virus/acquired immunodeficiency syndrome

Immune system: the bodily system that protects the body from foreign substances, cells, and tissues by producing an immune response

Incidence: the number of new cases of a particular disease

Isoniazid: one of the four first-line anti-TB antibiotics

Latent TB: a form of TB in which M. *tuberculosis* infection is present in the body but the immune system is keeping it in control and the person is not ill or infectious

Macrophage: a powerful white blood cell that functions as part of the immune system to help destroy foreign bodies such as bacteria and viruses

Mantoux test: the skin test that is used as a tool to diagnose TB in the United States

Microorganism: a microscopic or ultramicroscopic organism that is capable of response to stimuli, reproduction, growth, and mutation

Miliary TB: a form of TB with sudden onset and very rapid course of the illness, also known as "galloping" TB

Multidrug-resistant TB: a form of tuberculosis that is resistant to two or more of the primary drugs used for treatment

Mycobacterium: acid-fast aerobic bacterium of the Mycobacteriaceae family that is usually slender and difficult to stain; includes the causative agents of tuberculosis (M. *tuberculosis*)

Mycobacterium bovis (M. bovis): the type of mycobacterium that causes TB in cows

Mycobacterium tuberculosis (M. tuberculosis): the type of mycobacterium that causes tuberculosis in humans

Nucleic acid amplification (NAA) test: a diagnostic test to identify the presence of genetic information unique to M. *tuberculosis* directly in a preprocessed respiratory sample

Pathogenic: causing or capable of causing disease

Percussion: tapping the chest to produce sounds that give important information about the condition of the lungs

Phthisis: the name for TB used in ancient Greece and Rome

Prevalence: the proportion of a population with a specific condition at a designated time

Primary TB: active TB disease that develops immediately following infection

Pulmonary: relating to or associated with the lungs

Pyrazinamide: one of the four first-line anti-TB antibiotics

QuantiFERON®-TB Gold test (QFT-G): the blood test used to help diagnose TB infection

Rifampin: one of the four first-line anti-TB antibiotics

Sanatorium: a specialized health care facility that provides care for patients with TB

Scrofula: a form of TB that affects the lymph glands of the neck

Secondary TB: active TB disease that develops when TB bacteria reactivate after a period of being latent

Smear test: a diagnostic test; sputum is smeared on a glass slide and specially stained to permit identification of TB bacteria

Sputum: the matter discharged from the air passages in diseases of the lungs or upper respiratory tract that contains mucous and other products, including bacteria; for TB diagnosis, it is examined for the presence of TB bacteria during a smear or culture

Staining: a technique in which dye is used to color tissues or microorganisms so that they can be viewed more easily for examination

Streptomycin: the first antibiotic that effectively inhibited the growth of M. *tuberculosis* and had relatively low toxicity; discovered in 1943

T cell: a type of white blood cell involved in immune response

Treatment adherence: taking medication as prescribed for as long as necessary

Tubercle: a TB lesion that usually has a caseous necrosis center and consists of different types of cells and the products made by the disintegration of white blood cells and bacilli

Tubercle bacilli: the microorganisms that causes TB

Tuberculin: a sterile solution containing specific substances extracted from tubercle bacilli that is used in skin testing to diagnose TB

Tuberculosis (TB): a usually chronic, unpredictable disease that is caused by inhalation of airborne *Mycobacterium tuberculosis*; it most frequently affects the lungs and is characterized by fever, cough, difficulty in breathing, and the formation of tubercles

Bibliography

A roadmap for new tuberculosis drugs. *Lancet*. 2007;369(9575):1764.

Aagaard C, Dietrich J, Doherty M, Andersen P. TB vaccines: current status and future perspectives. *Immunol Cell Biol*. 2009;87(4):279–286.

Alisjahbana B, van Crevel R. Improved diagnosis of tuberculosis by better sputum quality. *Lancet*. 2007;369(9577):1908–1909.

American Lung Association. Tuberculosis. 2009. Available from: http://www.lungusa.org/atf/cf/%7B7a8d42c2-fcca-4604–8ade-7f5d5e762256%7D/ALA_LDD08_TB_FINAL.PDF.

Bartlett JG. Tuberculosis and HIV infection: partners in human tragedy. *J Infect Dis*. 2007;196 Suppl 1:S124–125.

Blanc FX, Havlir DV, Onyebujoh PC, Thim S, Goldfeld AE, Delfraissy JF. Treatment strategies for HIV-infected patients with tuberculosis: ongoing and planned clinical trials. *J Infect Dis*. 2007;196 Suppl 1:S46–51.

Blumberg HM, Burman WJ, Chaisson RE, Daley CL, Etkind SC, Friedman LN, et al. American Thoracic Society/Centers for Disease Control and Prevention/Infectious Diseases Society of America: treatment of tuberculosis. *Am J Respir Crit Care Med*. 2003;167(4):603–662.

Bonilla CA, Crossa A, Jave HO, Mitnick CD, Jamanca RB, Herrera C, et al. Management of extensively drug-resistant tuberculosis in Peru: cure is possible. *PLoS One*. 2008;3(8):e2957.

Borgdorff MW, Small PM. Scratching the surface of ignorance on MDR tuberculosis. *Lancet.* 2009;373(9678):1822–1824.

Brosch R, Vincent V. Cutting-edge science and the future of tuberculosis control. *Bulletin of the World Health Organization.* 2007;85 (5):410–412.

Cain KP, Benoit SR, Winston CA, Mac Kenzie WR. Tuberculosis among foreign-born persons in the United States. JAMA. 2008;300(4):405–412.

Campbell M. What tuberculosis did for modernism: the influence of a curative environment on modernist design and architecture. *Med Hist.* 2005;49(4): 463–488.

Center for Global Health Policy. Deadly Duo: The Synergy Between HIV/AIDS & Tuberculosis. June 2009. Available from http://www.idsociety.org/Work Area/showcontent.aspx?id=14756.

Centers for Disease Control and Prevention. Treatment of tuberculosis: American Thoracic Society, CDC, and Infectious Diseases Society of America. *Morbidity and Mortality Weekly Report.* June 20, 2003; 52(RR-11):1–71. Available from: http://www.cdc.gov/mmwr/preview/mmwrhtml/rr5211a1.htm.

Centers for Disease Control and Prevention. Controlling tuberculosis in the United States: recommendations from the American Thoracic Society, CDC, and the Infectious Disease Society of America. *Morbidity and Mortality Weekly Report.* November 4, 2005;54(RR12):1–81.

Centers for Disease Control and Prevention. TB and HIV/AIDS factsheet. January 2008. Available from: http://www.cdc.gov/hiv/resources/factsheets/PDF/hivtb.pdf.

Centers for Disease Control and Prevention. Trends in Tuberculosis—United States, 2007 *Morbidity and Mortality Weekly Report.* March 21, 2008;57(11): 281–285. Available from: http://www.cdc.gov/mmwr/preview/mmwrhtml/mm 5711a2.htm.

Centers for Disease Control and Prevention. World TB Day: partnerships for TB elimination. May 3, 2008. Available from: http://www.cdc.gov/tb/Worlf TBDay/default.htm.

Centers for Disease Control and Prevention, Division of Tuberculosis Elimination. Treatment of latent tuberculosis infection: maximizing adherence. 2005. Available from: http://www.cdc.gov/tb/publications/factsheets/treatment/LT BIadherence.pdf.

Centers for Disease Control and Prevention, Division of Tuberculosis Elimination. Treatment options for latent tuberculosis infection. April 2005. Available from: http://www.cdc.gov/tb/publications/factsheets/treatment/LTBItreatment options.htm.

Centers for Disease Control and Prevention, Division of Tuberculosis Elimination. Trends in tuberculosis incidence, 2006. March 23, 2007; 56(11):245–250. Available from: http://www.cdc.gov/mmwr/preview/mmwrhtml/mm5611a2.htm.

Centers for Disease Control and Prevention, Division of Tuberculosis Elimination. Treatment of latent tuberculosis infection (LTBI). July 2007. Available from: http://www.cdc.gov/tb/publications/factsheets/treatment/treatment LTBI.htm.

Centers for Disease Control and Prevention, Division of Tuberculosis Elimination. Quantiferon-TB Gold Test. October 2007. Available from: http://www.cdc.gov/tb/publications/factsheets/testing/QFT.htm.

Centers for Disease Control and Prevention, Division of Tuberculosis Elimination. Trends in tuberculosis—United States, 2008. *Morbidity and Mortality Weekly Report.* March 20, 2009;58(10):249–253. Available from: http://www.cdc.gov/mmwr/preview/mmwrhtml/mm5810a2.htm.

Centers for Disease Control and Prevention, Division of Tuberculosis Elimination. Questions and answers about TB. 2009. Available from: http://www.cdc.gov/tb/publications/faqs/pdfs/qa.pdf.

Centers for Disease Control and Prevention: The National Institute for Occupational Safety and Health. Infectious diseases: TB cases in the United States. *Evidence Package for the National Academies' Review.* 2006–2007.

Chalke HD. The impact of tuberculosis on history, literature and art. *Med Hist.* 1962;6(4):301–318.

Chan ED, Laurel V, Strand MJ, Chan JF, Huynh M-LN, Globe M, et al. Treatment and outcome analysis of 205 patients with multidrug-resistant tuberculosis. *Am J Respir Crit Care Med.* 2004;169:1103–1109.

Chhabria M, Jani M, Patel S. New frontiers in the therapy of tuberculosis: fighting with the global menace. *Mini Rev Med Chem.* 2009;9(4):401–430.

Churchyard GJ, Scano F, Grant AD, Chaisson RE. Tuberculosis preventive therapy in the era of HIV infection: overview and research priorities. *J Infect Dis.* 2007;196 Suppl 1:S52–62.

Cobelens FG, Heldal E, Kimerling ME, Mitnick CD, Podewils LJ, Ramachandran R, et al. Scaling up programmatic management of drug-resistant tuberculosis: a prioritized research agenda. *PLoS Med.* 2008;5(7):e150.

Connolly CA. *Saving Sickly Children: The Tuberculosis Preventorium in American Life, 1909–1970.* Piscataway, NJ: Rutgers University Press; 2008.

Daley CL. *Tuberculosis and Nontuberculous Mycobacterial Infections in Clinical Respiratory Medicine,* 3rd ed. Albert RK, Spiro, SG, Jett, JR, editors. Philadelphia, PA: Mosby; 2008.

Daniel TM. *Captain of Death: The Story of Tuberculosis.* Rochester, NY: University of Rochester Press; 1997.

Diacon AH, Pym A, Grobusch M, Patientia R, Rustomjee R, Page-Shipp L, et al. The diarylquinoline TMC207 for multidrug-resistant tuberculosis. *N Engl J Med.* 2009;360(23):2397–2405.

Dietrich J, Doherty TM. Interaction of Mycobacterium tuberculosis with the host: consequences for vaccine development. *APMIS*. 2009;117(5–6):440–457.

Dockrell HM, Zhang YA. courageous step down the road toward a new tuberculosis vaccine. *Am J Respir Crit Care Med*. 2009;179(8):628–629.

Dong K, Thabethe Z, Hurtado R, Sibaya T, Dlwati H, Walker B, et al. Challenges to the success of HIV and tuberculosis care and treatment in the public health sector in South Africa. *J Infect Dis*. 2007;196 Suppl 3:S491–496.

Dormandy T. *The White Death: A History of Tuberculosis*. New York, NY: Hambledon and London; 2001.

Dowdy DW, Chaisson RE, Maartens G, Corbett EL, Dorman SE. Impact of enhanced tuberculosis diagnosis in South Africa: a mathematical model of expanded culture and drug susceptibility testing. *Proc Natl Acad Sci USA*. 2008;105(32):11293–11298.

Dubois R, Dubois J. *The White Plague: Tuberculosis, Man, and Society*. Boston, MA: Little, Brown and Company; 1952.

Dye C, Harries AD, Maher D, Hosseini SM, Nkhoma W, Salaniponi FM *Disease and Mortality in Sub-Saharan Africa*. *Tuberculosis*, 2nd ed. Jamison DT, Feachem RG, Makgoba MW, Bos ER, Baingana FK, Hofman KJ, et al., editors. Washington, DC: World Bank Publications; 2006.

Fauci A, Kasper D, Braunwald E, Hauser S, Longo D, Jameson JL, et al. *Harrison's Principles of Internal Medicine*. New York, NY: McGraw Hill Companies; 2008. Available from: http://www.accessmedicine.com.

Financing the fight against AIDS, tuberculosis, and malaria. *Lancet*. 2007; 370(9594):1190.

Franke MF, Appleton SC, Bayona J, Arteaga F, Palacios E, Llaro K, et al. Risk factors and mortality associated with default from multidrug-resistant tuberculosis treatment. *Clin Infect Dis*. 2008;46(12):1844–1851.

Frieden TR. Lessons from tuberculosis control for public health. *Int J Tuberc Lung Dis*. 2009;13(4):421–428.

Friedland G, Churchyard GJ, Nardell E. Tuberculosis and HIV coinfection: current state of knowledge and research priorities. *J Infect Dis*. 2007;196 Suppl 1:S1–3.

Friedland G, Harries A, Coetzee D. Implementation issues in tuberculosis/HIV program collaboration and integration: 3 case studies. *J Infect Dis*. 2007;196 Suppl 1:S114–123.

Friedland JS. *Tuberculosis in Infectious Diseases*, 2nd ed. Cohen J, Powderly, WG, editors. Philadelphia, PA: Mosby; 2004.

Gandy M, Zulma A, eds. *The Return of the White Plague: Global Poverty and the "New" Tuberculosis*. New York, NY: Verso; 2003.

Global Tuberculosis Control 2009: Epidemiology, Strategy, Financing. Geneva, Switzerland: World Health Organization Press; 2009. Available from: http://www.who.int/tb/publications/global_report/2009/en/index.html.

Herzog H. History of tuberculosis. *Respiration*. 1998;65(1):5–15.

Hugonnet JE, Tremblay LW, Boshoff HI, Barry CE, 3rd, Blanchard JS. Meropenem-clavulanate is effective against extensively drug-resistant Mycobacterium tuberculosis. *Science*. 2009;323(5918):1215–1218.

Hung NV, Sy DN, Anthony RM, Cobelens FG, van Soolingen D. Fluorescence microscopy for tuberculosis diagnosis. *Lancet Infect Dis*. 2007;7(4):238–239; author reply 239–240.

Inge LD, Wilson JW. Update on the treatment of tuberculosis. *Am Fam Physician*. 2008;78(4):457–465.

Jasmer RM, Daley CL. Rifampin and pyrazinamide for treatment of latent tuberculosis infection: is it safe? *Am J Respir Crit Care Med*. 2003;167(6): 809–810.

Johnson JL, Jamil Hadad D, Dietze R, Maciel EL, Sewali B, Gitta P, et al. Shortening treatment in adults with non-cavitary tuberculosis and two-month culture conversion. *Am J Respir Crit Care Med*. 2009.

Kemp JR, Mann G, Nhlema Simwaka B, Salaniponi F, Squire S. Can Malawi's poor afford free tuberculosis services? Patient and household costs associated with a tuberculosis diagnosis in Lilongwe. *Bulletin of the World Health Organization*. 2007;85:580–585.

Khan MS, Dar O, Sismanidis C, Shah K, Godfrey-Faussett P. Improvement of tuberculosis case detection and reduction of discrepancies between men and women by simple sputum-submission instructions: a pragmatic randomised controlled trial. *Lancet*. 2007;369(9577):1955–1960.

Kidder T. *Mountains Beyond Mountains: The Quest of Paul Farmer, a Man Who Would Cure the World*. New York, NY: Random House; 2003.

Korenromp EL, Bierrenbach AL, Williams BG, Dye C. The measurement and estimation of tuberculosis mortality. *Int J Tuberc Lung Dis*. 2009;13(3):283–303.

Lee HSJ, editor. *Dates in Infectious Diseases: A Chronological Record of Progress in Infectious Diseases over the Last Millennium*. New York, NY: Parthenon Publishing Group; 2002.

Leung CC, Yew WW. Does current drug resistance surveillance provide useful information in tuberculosis? *Am J Respir Crit Care Med*. 2009;179(1):82; author reply 82–83.

Li X, Zhang Y, Shen X, Shen G, Gui X, Sun B, et al. Transmission of drug-resistant tuberculosis among treated patients in Shanghai, China. *J Infect Dis*. 2007;195(6):864–869.

LoBue P. Extensively drug-resistant tuberculosis. *Curr Opin Infect Dis*. 2009; 22(2):167–173.

LoBue P, Sizemore C, Castro KG. Centers for Disease Control and Prevention. Plan to combat extensively drug-resistant tuberculosis recommendations of the Federal Tuberculosis Task Force. *Morbidity and Mortality Weekly Report*.

February 13, 2009;58(RR03):1–43. Available from: http://www.cdc.gov/mmwr/preview/mmwrhtml/rr5803a1.htm?s_cid=rr5803a1_e.

Maartens G, Wilkinson RJ. Tuberculosis. *Lancet.* 2007;370(9604):2030–2043.

Mandell GL, Bennett, JE, Dolin, R. *Treatment of tuberculosis. Principles and Practice of Infectious Diseases*, 6th ed Philadelphia, PA: Churchill Livingstone; 2005.

Mant D, Mayon-White R. Tuberculosis: think globally and act locally. *Lancet.* 2007;369(9572):1493–1494.

Marais BJ, Graham SM, Cotton MF, Beyers N. Diagnostic and management challenges for childhood tuberculosis in the era of HIV. *J Infect Dis.* 2007;196 Suppl 1:S76–85.

Mayho P. *The Tuberculosis Survival Handbook,* 2nd ed. West Palm Beach, FL: Merit Publishing International; 2006.

Medpage Today. CDC urges nucleic acid amplification testing for all suspected TB. 2008. Available from: http://www.medpagetoday.com/InfectiousDisease/Tuberculosis/12465.

Mitnick CD, Appleton SC, Shin SS. Epidemiology and treatment of multidrug resistant tuberculosis. *Semin Respir Crit Care Med.* 2008;29(5):499–524.

Mitnick CD, Shin SS, Seung KJ, Rich ML, Atwood SS, Furin JJ, et al. Comprehensive treatment of extensively drug-resistant tuberculosis. *N Engl J Med.* 2008;359(6):563–574.

Moberg CL. *Rene Dubos, Friend of the Good Earth: Microbiologist, Medical Scientist, Environmentalist.* Washington, DC: ASM Press; 2005.

Murray & Nadel's Textbook of Respiratory Medicine, 4th ed. Tuberculosis. Mason RJ, Murray JF, Broaddus VC, Nadel JA, editors. Philadelphia, PA: Saunders Elsevier; 2005.

National Institute of Allergy and Infectious Disease. Tuberculosis (TB). 2009. Available from: http://www3.niaid.nih.gov/topics/tuberculosis/.

New Jersey Medical School. Global Tuberculosis Institute. History of TB. 2009. Available from: http://www.umdnj.edu/ntbcweb/tbhistory.htm.

New York City Department of Health and Mental Hygiene: Bureau of Tuberculosis Control. Rapid diagnostic tests for tuberculosis. 2009. Available from: http://www.nyc.gov/html/doh/html/tb/tb1g.shtml.

Nuermberger E, Mitchison DA. Once-weekly treatment of tuberculosis with the diarylquinoline R207910: a real possibility. *Am J Respir Crit Care Med.* 2009;179(1):2–3.

Nyendak MR, Lewinsohn DA, Lewinsohn DM. New diagnostic methods for tuberculosis. *Curr Opin Infect Dis.* 2009;22(2):174–182.

Oliver P. *Blues Fell This Morning,* 2nd ed. Cambridge, UK: Cambridge University Press; 1990.

Onyebujoh PC, Ribeiro I, Whalen CC. Treatment Options for HIV-Associated Tuberculosis. *J Infect Dis.* 2007;196 Suppl 1:S35–45.

Pai M, Kalantri S, Dheda K. New tools and emerging technologies for the diagnosis of tuberculosis: part I. Latent tuberculosis. *Expert Rev Mol Diagn.* 2006;6(3):413–422.

Perkins MD, Cunningham J. Facing the crisis: improving the diagnosis of tuberculosis in the HIV era. *J Infect Dis.* 2007;196 Suppl 1:S15–27.

Porco TC, Getz WM. Controlling extensively drug-resistant tuberculosis. *Lancet.* 2007;370(9597):1464–1465.

Potter P. On the threshold of illness and emotional isolation [about the cover]. May 2006. Available from: http://www.cdc.gov/ncidod/EID/vol12no05/about_cover.htm.

Prideaux S. *Edvard Munch: Behind the Scream.* New Haven, CT: Yale University Press; 2007.

Radosevic K, Rodriguez A, Lemckert A, Goudsmit J. Heterologous prime-boost vaccinations for poverty-related diseases: advantages and future prospects. *Expert Rev Vaccines.* 2009;8(5):577–592.

Rieder HL. Fourth-generation fluoroquinolones in tuberculosis. *Lancet.* 2009;373(9670):1148–1149.

Ringold S, Lynm C, Glass RM. JAMA patient page. Tuberculosis. *JAMA.* 2008;300(4):464.

Rodriguez GM. Control of iron metabolism in Mycobacterium tuberculosis. *Trends Microbiol.* 2006;14(7):320–327.

Rothman SM. *Living in the Shadow of Death: Tuberculosis and the Social Experience of Illness in American History.* Baltimore, MD: Johns Hopkins University Press; 1995.

Ryan F. *The Forgotten Plague: How the Battle against Tuberculosis Was Won—And Lost.* Boston, MA: Back Bay Books; 1994.

Ryan F. *Tuberculosis: The Greatest Story Never Told.* Sheffield, UK: Swift Publishers Ltd; 1992.

Seigworth GR. Early practice: bloodletting over the centuries. The Educational Broadcasting Corporation; 2002. Available from: http://www.pbs.org/wnet/redgold/basics/bloodlettinghistory.html.

Shah NS, Pratt R, Armstrong L, Robison V, Castro KG, Cegielski JP. Extensively drug-resistant tuberculosis in the United States, 1993–2007. *JAMA.* 2008;300(18):2153–2160.

Shenoi S, Heysell S, Moll A, Friedland G. Multidrug-resistant and extensively drug-resistant tuberculosis: consequences for the global HIV community. *Curr Opin Infect Dis.* 2009;22(1):11–17.

Sleigh AC. Health-system reforms to control tuberculosis in China. *Lancet.* 2007;369(9562):626–627.

Spigelman MK. New tuberculosis therapeutics: a growing pipeline. *J Infect Dis.* 2007;196 Suppl 1:S28–34.

Starke JR, Jacobs, RF. Tuberculosis. *Principles and Practice of Pediatric Infectious Diseases.* 3rd ed. Long SS, editor. Philadelphia, PA: Churchill Livingstone; 2008.

Stephenson J. IOM report a blueprint for elimination of TB. *JAMA.* 2000; 283:2776–2777.

Stop TB Partnership. Stop TB News: Stop TB ambassador appointed: Figo's new goal is fighting tuberculosis. 2008. Available from: http://www.stoptb.org/ resource_center/assets/documents/StopTBNewsJanuary2008.pdf.

Targeted tuberculin testing and treatment of latent tuberculosis infection. *Am J Respir Crit Care Med.* 2000;161(4 Pt 2):S221–247.

Todar K. *University of Wisconsin Online Textbook of Bacteriology. Tuberculosis.* 2008. Available from: http://www.textbookofbacteriology.net/tuberculosis.html

U.S. Centers for Disease Control and Prevention. The body: the complete HIV/Aids resource. Nucleic acid amplification tests for diagnosis of tuberculosis. 1996. Available from: http://www.thebody.com/content/treat/art17232. html?ts=pf.

Vitoria M, Granich R, Gilks CF, Gunneberg C, Hosseini M, Were W, et al. The global fight against HIV/AIDS, tuberculosis, and malaria: current status and future perspectives. *Am J Clin Pathol.* 2009;131(6):844–848.

Waksman SA. JBC centennial, 1905–2005. 100 years of biochemistry and molecular biology: Selman Waksman: the father of antibiotics. *J Biol Chem.* 2004;279(48):e7.

Wang JY, Lee LN, Lai HC, Hsu HL, Liaw YS, Hsueh PR, et al. Prediction of the tuberculosis reinfection proportion from the local incidence. *J Infect Dis.* 2007;196(2):281–288.

Wang L, Liu J, Chin DP. Progress in tuberculosis control and the evolving public-health system in China. *Lancet.* 2007;369(9562):691–696.

Wood R. The case for integrating tuberculosis and HIV treatment services in South Africa. *J Infect Dis.* 2007;196 Suppl 3:S497–499.

Woods GL. Molecular methods in the detection and identification of mycobacterial infections. *Arch Pathol Lab Med.* 1999;123(11):1002–1006.

World Health Organization. Guidelines for social mobilization: a human rights approach to tuberculosis. 2001. Available from: http://www.stoptb.org/events/ world_tb_day/2001/H.RightsReport2001.pdf.

World Health Organization (press release, March 23, 2001). Bill & Melinda Gates Foundation awards $10 million to develop new diagnostics for tuberculosis. 2001. Available from: http://www.who.int/inf-pr-2001/en/pr2001–15.html.

World Health Organization (press release). WHO reports 10 million TB patients successfully treated under "DOTS" 10 years after declaring TB a global emergency. 2003. Available from: http://www.who.int/mediacentre/news/releases/2003/pr25/en/.

World Health Organization. Anti-tuberculosis drug-resistance in the world. Report No. 4.; 2008. Available from: http://www.who.int/tb/publications/2008/drs_report4_26feb08.pdf.

World Health Organization. The five elements of DOTS. 2008. Available from: http://www.who.int/tb/dots/whatisdots/en/index.html.

World Health Organization. Global tuberculosis control 2009: Epidemiology, strategy, financing. Geneva, Switzerland: WHO Press; 2009. Available from: http://www.who.int/tb/publications/global_report/2009/en/index.html.

World Health Organization. Global tuberculosis control: key points. 2009. Available from: www.who.int/tb/publications/global_report/2009/key_points/.

World Health Organization. TB/HIV FACTS 2009. Available from: http://www.who.int/tb/challenges/hiv/factsheet_hivtb_2009.pdf.

World Health Organization and The Stop TB Strategy. Building on and enhancing DOTS to meet the TB-related Millennium Development Goals. 2006. Available from: http://www.who.int/tb/publications/2006/stop_tb_strategy.pdf.

World Health Organization and The Stop TB Stategy. Components of the Stop TB Strategy. 2006. Available from: http://www.who.int/tb/stratgy/stop_tb_strategy/en/index.html.

World Health Organization and The Stop TB Partnership. World TB Day—March 24th. 2009. Available from: http://www.stoptb.org/events/world_tb_day/.

Wright A, Zignol M, Van Deun A, Falzon D, Gerdes SR, Feldman K, et al. Epidemiology of antituberculosis drug resistance 2002–07: an updated analysis of the Global Project on Anti-Tuberculosis Drug Resistance Surveillance. *Lancet*. 2009.

Yew WW, Leung CC. Management of multidrug-resistant tuberculosis: update 2007. *Respirology*. 2008;13(1):21–46.

Yew WW, Leung CC. Update in tuberculosis 2007. *Am J Respir Crit Care Med*. 2008;177(5):479–485.

Index

About the Author

CAROL A. DYER, MS, ELS, is a science writer and board certified editor in the life sciences. She is a senior medical writer at Prescott Medical Communications Group in Chicago, Illinois. In addition, Carol works as a freelance science writer exploring topics of interest in the fields of science and medicine.